Intermittent Fasting Guide For Women Over 50

2 Books In 1

Learn To Lose Weight, Detox Your Body, Increase Longevity And Improve Well-Being With The Method That's Right For You (16: 8, 5:2, 12:12).

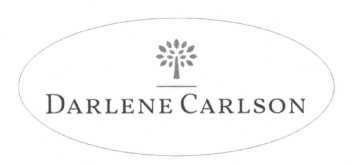

DARLENE CARLSON

Thank you for purchasing the book,

after reading it, I would be grateful if you could take a minute of your time to leave an honest Amazon review about my work and share your experience with other customers.

Thank you!

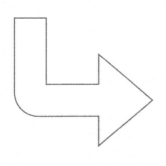 

Contents

Introduction

M ore than half the entire population of the world is overweight. Think about that for just a second – it is alarming how quickly the prevalence of obesity and overweight has grown in just the last 30 years or so. This increasing trend of obesity and people who are overweight has also led to the dieting and supplement industry exploiting this as an opportunity for them to gain billions in profit – often promoting products that are worthless and ineffective when it comes to losing excess fat that has been stored in the body.

For long-term weight loss, there are techniques that have been shown to be successful. You will be able to safely lose weight when you follow a well-planned strategy (losing weight too fast is harmful) and you will be able to maintain that weight for years to come, as long as you make sure you eat a healthy diet. Habits of lifestyles and moving on.

Intermittent fasting is a technique that relies on fasting for a period of time and then having a relatively small dining room window, where all the meals for the day should be placed.

The reason you have taken this book is probably because you have tried many diets and found that the success rate is often not something you want. That's true, most of the diets out there fail. Many of these diets not only fail, but cause problems as soon as you stop watching the show. For many people, weight gain is a very unpleasant complication after going on a diet plan.

You have probably heard of intermittent fasting and that it has had positive effects on thousands of people in the past. Scientific evidence has already shown this. However, you are not sure how to start, where to start, when to eat, what schedule to follow, and of course what to eat.

Continue reading to know more about intermittent fasting!

Chapter 1. What Is Intermittent Fasting?

B asically, fasting is defined as abstaining from eating anything. It is the deliberate action of depriving the body of any form of food for more than six hours, whereas intermittent fasting is one of its forms where the fast is carried out in a cyclic manner with the aim to reduce the overall caloric intake in a day. To most people, it may sound unhealthy and damaging for the body, but scientific research has proven that fasting can produce positive results on the human mind and body. It teaches self-discipline and fights against bad eating practices. It is basically an umbrella term that is used to define all voluntary forms of fasting. This dietary approach does not restrict the consumption of certain food items; rather, it works by reducing the overall food intake, leaving enough space to meet the essential nutrients the body needs. Therefore, it is proven to be far more effective and much easier in implementation, given that the dieter completely understands the nature and science of intermittent fasting.

Intermittent fasting is categorized into three broad methods of food abstinence, including the alternate day fasting, daily restrictions, and periodic fasting. The means may vary, but the end goal of intermittent fasting remains the same, that is to achieve a better metabolism, healthy body weight, and active lifestyle. The American Heart Association, AHA, has also studied intermittent fasting and its results. According to the AHA, it can help in countering insulin resistance, cardiometabolic diseases, and leads to weight loss. However, a question mark remains on the sustainability of this health effective method. The 2019 research "Effects of intermittent fasting on health, aging, and disease" has also found intermittent fasting to be effective against insulin resistance, inflammation, hypertension, obesity, and dyslipidemia. However, the work on this dietary approach is still underway, and the traditional methods of fasting which existed for almost the entire human history, in every religion from Buddhism to Jainism, Orthodox Christianity, Hinduism, and Islam, are studied to found relevance in today's age of science and technology.

How Does It Work

Intermittent fasting works between alternating periods of eating and fasting. It is a much more flexible approach, as there are many options to choose from according to body type, size, weight goals, and nutritional needs. The human body works like a synchronized machine that requires sufficient time for self-healing and repair. When we constantly eat junk and unhealthy food without the consideration of our caloric needs, it leads to obesity and toxic build-up in the body. That is why fasting comes as a natural means of detoxifying the body and providing it enough time to utilize its fat deposits.

Whatever the human body consumes is ultimately broken into glucose, which is later utilized by the cells in glycolysis to release energy. As the blood glucose level rises, insulin is produced to lower the levels and allow the liver to carry out De Novo Lipogenesis, the process in which the excess glucose is turned into glycogen and ultimately stored into fat, resulting in obesity. Intermittent fasting seems to reverse this process by deliberately creating energy deprivation, which is then fulfilled by breaking down the existing fat deposits.

Intermittent fasting works through lipolysis; though it is a natural body process, it can only be initiated when the blood glucose levels drop to a sufficiently low point. That point can be achieved through fasting and exercising. When a person cuts off the external glucose supply for several hours, the body switches to lipolysis. This process of breaking the fats also releases other by-products like ketones which are capable of reducing the oxidative stress of the body and help in its detoxification.

Mark Mattson, a neuroscientist from the Johns Hopkins Medicine University, has studied intermittent fasting for almost 25 years of his career. He laid out the workings of intermittent fasting by clarifying its clinical application and the science behind it. According to him, intermittent fasting must be opted for a healthy lifestyle.

While discussing the application of this dietary approach, it is imperative to understand how intermittent fasting stands out from casual dieting practices. It is not mere abstinence from eating. What is eaten in this dietary lifestyle is equally important as the fasting itself. It does not result in malnutrition; rather, it promotes healthy eating along with the fast. Intermittent fasting is divided into two different states that follow one another. The cycle starts with the "FED" state, which is followed by a "Fasting" state. The duration of the fasting state and the frequency of the FED state are established by the method of intermittent fasting. The latter is characterized by high blood glucose levels, whereas during the fasting state the body goes through a gradual decline in glucose levels. This decline in glucose signals the pancreas and the brain to meet the body's energy needs by processing the available fat molecules. However, if the fasting state is followed by a FED state in which a person binge eats food rich in Carbs and fats, it will turn out to be more hazardous for their health. Therefore, the fasting period must be accompanied by a healthy diet.

The Science Behind Intermittent Fasting

Biologically, intermittent fasting works at many levels, from cellular levels to gene expression and body growth. In order to understand the science behind the workings of intermittent fasting, it is important to learn about the role of insulin levels, human growth hormone, cellular repair, and gene expression. Intermittent fasting firstly lowers the glucose levels, which in turn drops the insulin levels. This lowering of insulin helps fat burning in the body, thus gradually curbing obesity and related disorders. Controlled levels of insulin are also responsible for preventing diabetes and insulin resistance. On the other hand, intermittent fasting boosts the production of human growth hormones up to five times. The increased production of HGH aids quick fat burning and muscle formation.

During the fasting state, the body goes into the process of self-healing at cellular levels, thus removing the unwanted, unfunctional cells and debris. This creates a cleansing effect that directly or indirectly nourishes the body and allows it to grow under reduced oxidative stress. Likewise, fasting even affects the gene expression within the human body. The cell functions according to the coding and decoding of the gene's expression; when this transcription occurs at a normal pace in a healthy environment, it automatically translates into the longevity of the cells, and fasting ensures unhindered transcription. Thus, intermittent fasting fights aging, cancer, and boosts the immune system by strengthening the body cells.

Chapter 2. Pros And Cons

Y ou will find cons and pros to every lifestyle. For example, when you're eating a nutritious and healthy diet, you might lose weight and gain health but cannot eat all the favorite foods of yours in the amount you'd like. On the other hand, when you eat junk food all the time you may enjoy yourself, but you will lose health and gain weight. In the same way, there are naturally both pros and cons to intermittent fasting, and by understanding what they are, you can better manage your lifestyle. Like all things, you will find that these pros and cons are most evened out when intermittent fasting is moderated. If a person only rarely practices fasting, then they will, in turn, only experience a few of the benefits. On the other hand, if they practice intermittent fasting overly enthusiastically and longer periods than healthy, they will experience more of the drawbacks.

Thankfully, with a balanced intermittent fasting schedule, you can find yourself experiencing many benefits and few, if any, of the drawbacks.

While some pros and cons of intermittent fasting are universal, others can be affected by gender and age. In this chapter, we will be exploring what pros and cons you individually may experience as a woman in or over her fifties.

Pros

Boost Weight Loss

Most people discover intermittent fasting either because they want to lose weight or gain health benefits. But, sometimes losing weight can accomplish both of those simultaneously, as a high body fat percentage can increase high blood pressure, cholesterol, and early mortality. Whether you are hoping to gain these health benefits by losing weight or wish to lose weight to feel more comfortable in your skin, you will love the way that intermittent fasting can boost your weight loss.

Balance Important Hormones

Thankfully, studies have found intermittent fasting can help balance a person's cortisol and melioration levels. It does this in a variety of ways. For instance, it can help to reduce cortisol by balancing and regulating blood sugar levels. Balancing cortisol sets off a chain reaction that improves the balance of other hormones, including melatonin. One simple change can benefit many hormones and systems within your body.

Improve Heart Health

As we age, we all must take even more care of our heart health. After all, heart disease is the number one killer of both men and women. While most often doctors educate men on the symptoms and warning signs of heart attacks, women are often forgotten, leading to increased risk of death. This means women must be extra vigilant, taking care of their heart health and educating themselves on the warning signs of heart attacks.

One crucial way to increase heart health is to watch your cholesterol. There is not a single type of cholesterol, but several. The two main types include LDL, known as the "bad" cholesterol, and HDL, known as the "good" cholesterol. While LDL cholesterol will increase your risk of heart attack and heart disease, HDL cholesterol will protect your heart and remove LDL cholesterol from your body.

Increase Mental Energy and Efficiency

We all need mental energy to get through the day. When our mind is sluggish, we are unable to think, accomplish anything, and sometimes we may be unable even to stay awake. We have all had troubles focusing on work, completing a math problem, remembering what we have read, and so on. This is all due to a lack of mental energy and efficiency. You may think that intermittent fasting would further reduce your mental state, as hunger makes focusing difficult, but the opposite is exact.

Reduce the Potential Risk of Developing Cancer

Of course, nobody can promise that any lifestyle choice will prevent you from developing cancer. However, studies have found that intermittent fasting can potentially reduce your risk. Further studies are ongoing, but current research through animal studies have proven promising. For instance, it was found that rats with tumors survive longer when placed on fasting schedules than the control group.

Increase Longevity

Early studies on animals have found that by including intermittent fasting, an animal can experience an increased lifespan. These studies found that even if animals had a higher body fat percentage than the control group, including intermittent fasting, they were able to increase their lifespan and longevity.

This makes sense, as intermittent fasting has many health benefits, and when all of these benefits are compounded together, it naturally results in a longer lifespan.

Lifestyle Ease

We all want improving health and weight, but it is important also to have an easier lifestyle. When it is difficult to gain health and weight, many of us fail, as life is already busy and difficult enough without adding added worry and tasks. If a person cooks more, eat more frequently, and always worry about a diet, they are unlike to stick to it, as it is merely unmaintainable.

It supports the secretion of the growth hormone.

It's present in kids more than in grown-ups, but it still helps a lot. The growth hormone decreases fat and improves the development of bone and muscles. It does this by turning glycogen to glucose into the bloodstream. This enables fat burn without the reduction of muscles. When you sleep and exercise enough, the growth hormone is also boosted.

It enables you to avoid heart illnesses.

Both blood glucose control and fat loss are done by IF improve heart health. The likelihood of getting coronary artery heart illness can also be reduced.

Intermittent fasting is very versatile and can fit in any schedule.

It is not as challenging as certain diets that unnecessarily trigger a huge disturbance in your life. There is no particular time to perform the IF. They can be blended as you think it is appropriate for your timetable. You are not boxed into any regiment that you cannot retain easily. Intermittent rapidity adapts to life's unpredictability. This can also be practiced everywhere globally as there is no special gear you need to do it; it only restricts your feeding and is therefore much easier and more practical than many diets. It's completely all right, even if you have to halt fasting for a while. In a matter of minutes, you can begin fasting again.

It accepts all food

Organic foods have more nutrients than processed foods. These organic products are unfortunately quite costly, so purchasing them will diminish your pockets every day. They can be almost 10 times more expensive than processed products. It is easier to afford processed products as they are cheap. No matter the effectiveness of a diet, if you can't afford it, it cannot help you. Fasting is in the first position of cost-effectiveness since it is completely free. You don't have to purchase any meals, so it costs you no cash. There's no reason you purchase costly meals or supplements or any drug that makes it cheap for all.

Simple to practice

Intermediate fasting is easy to do and doesn't have any complicated scheduling, it is quite direct. This causes it to be simpler to pursue and more efficient than many diets.

Opens up your mind

It enables you to regulate your mental procedures as IF opens up your body. You are used to responding to your body's urges because you consume whenever you feel slightly hungry. You are released from the control of your body as a result of practicing IF.

Corrects insulin resistance

This is the simplest and easiest route to reduce insulin resistance and insulin levels. It has a highly effective impact. It works better than a rigid low Carbs diet.

Improves your metabolism

Intermittent fasting enhances your metabolism by considerably reducing the number of calories you eat in one day. During the feeding time you have, it is almost possible to eat the suggested daily calorific requirements. This causes modifications in the body and fat burning. It also helps you burn fat, even if you eat the normal calories your system requires, as it will make you burn fat for power instead of Carbs.

Cons

Getting Started Takes an Adjustment

Any lifestyle change takes an adjustment, and it can take months for something to become a habit. Naturally, intermittent fasting is quite an adjustment for people who are used to grazing on food throughout the day. This means that if you push yourself to go into an advanced version of intermittent fasting when you first begin, you can become overwhelmed. But if you start slowly and allow your body to adjust in its own time, you will find it happens much more naturally and becomes easy to stick to.

Potential to Overeat

While intermittent fasting should naturally reduce caloric intake, if a person pushes themselves to fast when they are overly hungry, it might lead to overeating during their eating window. This is because the person feels hungry for so long when fasting when they finally eat their body and believes it must make up for the calories it missed. The result is that the person either hits a weight loss plateau or even experience increased weight.

Possible Leptin Imbalance

The hormone leptin is important as it signals to your body that you are full have no longer need to eat. But when a person practices intermittent fasting, it may temporarily disrupt this hormone's production. However, this is usually only a short-term problem, and once a person's body adjusts to their fasting and eating windows, their leptin will balance itself out. Typically, a leptin imbalance is only a real problem when a person dives head-first into intermittent fasting and attempt to practice advanced level fasting when they are still only a beginner.

You May Become Dehydrated

Many people do not drink enough water. In general, doctors recommend that we drink half of our body's weight in pounds in ounces of water. This means that if you weigh two-hundred pounds, you should be drinking one-hundred ounces of water daily.

Lots of people don't drink water that is enough as it's, but this can make dehydration worse when an individual is practicing fasting. This is because fasting boosts the metabolism, and when your cells are in a metabolic accelerated state, they require more water for fuel. If you are not giving them enough water during periods of fasting, you can quickly become dehydrated. Not only that but when fasting, you are likely to lose a lot of water weight, which can result in dehydration and a deficiency in electrolytes. Make sure that you not only drink plenty of water but also consume enough electrolytes to prevent this. Thankfully, dehydration is easy to avoid if you remain proactive.

Not Everyone Can Practice Intermittent Fasting

Intermittent fasting is a beautiful and healthy lifestyle for the general population. After all, the human body is designed for practice periods of fasting naturally. However, not every person can practice fasting. Some people, due to chronic illness, may be unable to participate. Ultimately, you must ask your doctor if you are healthy enough to practice short-term fasting.

It can trigger the re-feeding syndrome

This is a hazardous and fatal disorder that can happen if you suffer from malnutrition. It is when electrolyte and liquid imbalances occur when malnourished individuals have been hospitalized for a long time and eat again after a long time. The chance of acquiring re-feeding syndrome increases when bodily weight is very small and not eating for more than ten days.

Having low energy

Although after a while starvation passes, life isn't predictable. You can take part in a tiresome activity that makes you hungry and ultimately unproductive until the hunger goes, or you eat. You may have been used to eating a bunch of snacks during the day and quit instantly due to fasting, which may cause a few side-effects. These side effects involve headaches, bad temper, lack of power, constipation, and low concentration levels. It may also decrease your motivation. This sort of fasting can have an adverse fitness effect if you have a health condition. It is not suitable for all. For example, hypoglycemic people require glucose all day, so they can't profit from fasting.

Interfere with the social side of eating

Eating from ancient times was a significant social event. Special times, festivities, milestone accomplishment and other activities require meal sharing with your friends. IF can mess with your personal life when you change your routine which may not correspond to the regular eating schedule. During occasions where everyone eats and eats, you may stand out as the one who does not want to participate. Many activities including dinner meetings, family meals, and romantic meals are missed among many others.

Reproductive complications in some women

If the fasting is carried out in a fashion that mainly restricts Carbs and Protein, it can trigger fertility problems in females, lead to electrolyte defects and trigger nutritional deficits. There are also long-term adverse health effects. Intermediate fasting is linked to menstrual, premature menopause and health problems. Research indicates that ovary size can be reduced, thus influencing reproduction and decreasing bodily volume.

Digestive complications

It can lead to problems linked to digestion. When food is eaten too rapidly, a large meal may cause digestive problems. People who tend to have larger dishes during the feeding period digest them for a longer period. It increases the pressure on your digestive system, triggering indigestion and bloating. This will have a stronger impact on people with weak guts.

Weight regains

Intermittent acceleration reduces the body's reliance on carbohydrates for fuel and decreases fat dependency for power. There is an improvement in the decomposition of stored fats. The body undergoes physiological changes as a reaction to a drastic decrease in the body's power consumption. This implies that you might not be in a position to keep the weight of yours or perhaps even gain more weight despite extreme dietary restrictions.

Having seen the strengths and downsides of this fasting protocol, it is evident that each benefit's amount and weight is more advantageous than the downsides. Intermittent fasting will greatly improve the quality and the quantity of your life without a doubt.

Chapter 3. Different Types of Intermittent Fasting

I n order to harness and manipulate autophagy to benefit your body, you need to be able to upregulate its functioning within your cells. There are various ways to do this, and we will look at these ways, as well as how they work so that you can better understand how they work to affect your body. By upregulating autophagy, you are able to make your body resistant to many diseases.

Water Fasting

The first type of fasting we will look at is water fasting. Water fasting is a method of fasting in which a person does not ingest anything except water for a period of time. Many people practice water fasting for periods up to 72 hours, but this is a decision that should be made with the help of a doctor.

If you have ever gone into the hospital for a medical procedure, they likely told you that you could not eat food and could only drink water for a certain amount of time before the procedure. This practice would have been a form of water fasting. Some people also try water fasting as a method of "detoxing" their bodies. Another use for it though is to induce autophagy manually. Many people practice periods of water fasting to induce autophagy in order to rid their body of potentially harmful viruses or bacteria in an effort to reduce their risk of diseases such as cancer and Alzheimer's and even increase their lifespan. This is because of the cleansing properties of autophagy, as it breaks down infected cells and uses their salvageable parts for new and healthy cells to be generated. Autophagy can reduce the risk of cancers because of the way that it clears the body of damaged cells, which could otherwise accumulate and develop into cancer.

There are added benefits of water fasting that do not directly involve autophagy, but that is worth noting anyway. Water fasting has been shown to reduce blood pressure, cholesterol and even improve the functioning of insulin in the body, therefore improving blood sugar.

The problem with water fasting is that it can be quite dangerous if not practiced in a safe and monitored way. Consult a doctor before attempting a water fast so that you can ensure you are doing so in a safe way. There are some groups of people who should not practice water fasting. These groups include pregnant women, children, the elderly, and people with eating disorders.

Another thing to keep in mind when attempting a water fast in an effort to lose weight is that the weight lost during a water fast may not be the exact type of weight that you are trying to lose. During a water fast, there is a severe restriction in calories, which leads to the breakdown of fat stores, but some of the weight loss could also include water weight, stored carbohydrates and sometimes muscle (in longer fasts). What this means is that after a water fast, the weight loss may come back quite quickly if the majority was water or carbohydrate stores, as these are replenished very quickly once a person begins eating again. If this is the case, do not be concerned, this is a very normal reaction for your body to have as it is built to anticipate unexpected fasts and therefore has ways to protect you from these, such as storing carbohydrates.

When approaching a water fast, it is beneficial to prepare your body for a few days leading up to it by tapering off your eating portions in order to remove food from your day gradually. This will better prepare your body to go without food for a day or two. Another way to get your body prepared to water fast is to fast for part of the day so that it can get accustomed to spending some time without food. You may also be wondering how a water fast could make you lose water weight, but it is entirely possible and even likely. This is because much of the water we bring into our bodies throughout the day is enclosed in the foods we eat. If your water intake remains the same, but your food ingestion dramatically decreases, you could end up becoming dehydrated and thus losing water weight.

You will also need to adjust your activities to accommodate this water fast, especially if it is your first time trying it. If you are not used to fasting, you may feel dizzy or light-headed, and this may make some of your daily tasks more difficult. This could be due to lower blood sugar or lower blood pressure if you are dehydrated. Be sure to keep this in mind as you attempt a water fast and be sure to increase your water intake to avoid a drop in blood pressure.

There is still much more research that needs to be done surrounding water fasting in humans in particular. Water fasting as a method of weight loss is a relatively new approach and one that is just beginning to be explored with human test subjects.

16 And 8

This is the method where you would eat for 8 hours of the day and fast for 16 hours. When doing this method of IF, you would usually skip breakfast and eat between the hours of 1pm and 9pm, or 12 noon and 8pm. The hours you choose can vary depending on your work schedule and your lifestyle, but the key is that you eat for 8 hours of the day and have a longer portion of the day in which you are fasting. This is the most popular method of IF and is the easiest if you are new to following specific diets. Many people will naturally eat during an 8-hour window of the day if they do not tend to eat breakfast, which is why this method is the easiest to transition to. Some people prefer to use different ranges of hours, but in terms of research, 16 and 8 has been shown to be the most effective. If you are looking for something a little different, we will look at the two next most common methods below.

5:2

This method is different from the other two in that it involves a number of calories instead of hours. However, similar to the previous method, you are breaking up your week into different days instead of breaking up your day into hours.

In this method, you will restrict your caloric intake to between 500 and 600 calories on two days of the week. This is similar to the Eat-Stop-Eat method, except that instead of fully fasting on Monday and Thursday (for example), you will greatly restrict your caloric intake. For the other five days of the week, you will eat as you normally would. This is a method of intermittent eating, though it does not involve complete fasting. This method would be good for those who are unable to fast for two days of the week completely but who want to try a form of intermittent eating still. For example, this would be a good option for someone who works a physically laborious job and who cannot be feeling light-headed during the workday.

Eat-Stop-Eat

This method is a little different than the 16 and 8 method, as instead of breaking the day up into hours, you would be breaking your week up into days. You would fast for either one or two days of the week, not on back-to-back days. For example, you would fast from after lunch on Monday until after lunch on Tuesday and then again beginning after lunch on Thursday. For all the other days of the week, you could eat normally as you wish. This type is similar to water fasting in that it is a period of time where you are fasting, which is 24 hours in length. However, it is intermittent in that it only lasts 24 hours and repeats itself twice every week consistently. A water fast could be a one-off for 72 hours.

With this method, you will have to keep in mind that what you choose to eat and in what quantities on the days that you are not fasting will have effects on the results you see. You want to ensure you are not bingeing on the days that you are not fasting. This method is a good choice for those who prefer more flexibility during their eating times and do not want to restrict their eating to a small 8-hour window of the day, namely those who want to eat breakfast. This could be good for those who have longer working days and who prefer to have a longer time to eat during the day.

Alternate Day Fasting

This method of fasting involves fasting every other day and eating normally on the non-fasting days. Similar to other forms of IF, you are able to drink as much as you want of calorie-free drinks such as black coffee, tea, and water. You would fast for 24 hours on your fasting days, for example, from before dinner on one day until before dinner the next day. This method can be very successful or very unsuccessful depending on the person. The problem with this method is that it can lead to bingeing on the non-fasting days. If, however, you are a person that does not tend to binge, you may enjoy the flexibility that this diet offers by allowing you to eat whatever you want on alternating days.

There is a modification that some people choose to apply to this form of IF, where they allow themselves to eat 500 calories on their fasting days. This works out to about 20-25% of an adult person's daily energy needs, which will still put you in an extreme calorie deficit for those days, leading to the induction of autophagy. This method allows a person to continue with this diet consistently for a longer period of time than they may be able to with full fasts. It has the same effectiveness and works better with our modern lifestyles.

This type of IF has been shown to be very beneficial for weight loss and is a good choice for those who have weight loss as their main priority. Because of the calorie deficit that it put a person into, they are using more energy than they are putting into their body, which leads to a breakdown of fat stores and weight loss.

Women-Specific Methods of Intermittent Fasting

There is some evidence that suggests that Intermittent Fasting affects the bodies of men and women differently. The bodies of women are much more sensitive to small calorie changes, especially small negative changes in the intake of calories. Since the bodies of women are made for conceiving and growing babies, women's bodies must be sensitive to any sort of changes that may occur in the internal environment of the body to a larger degree than the bodies of men, in order to ensure that it will produce healthy and strong progeny. For this reason, however, some women may have trouble practicing intermittent fasting according to the above methods. These methods may involve too much restriction for the body of a woman, and she may feel some negative effects such as light-headedness or fatigue. In order to prevent this, there are some adjusted methods of intermittent fasting that will work better for women's bodies. This is not to say that women cannot practice IF or fasting of any sort, but that they must keep this in mind when deciding to try a fasting diet. Women can take a modified approach to fasting so that the internal environment of their bodies remains healthy. There are some slightly different patterns of IF that may be safer and more beneficial for women. We will look at these below.

Crescendo

This method is quite similar to the Eat-Stop-Eat method, except that in this one, the hours have been changed slightly. This fasting regimen involves breaking up the week into days as well as breaking up the days into hours. In this case, the woman would fast for 14 to 16 hours of the day twice a week and eating normally every other day. These fasting days would not be back-to-back and would not be more than twice per week.

Alternate Day 5:2

Alternatively, she could fast every other day but only for 12-14 hours, eating normally on the days in between. On the fasting days, she would eat 25% of her normal calorie intake, making it a reduction in calories and not a full-blown fast.

14 and 10

In this method, the day would be broken up into segments of hours. The woman would fast for 14 hours of the day and eat for 10 hours. Beginning with this modified version will allow her body to become used to fasting. Eventually, when she is comfortable with it, she can change the hours by one hour per day in order to reach 16 and 8.

By reducing the hours of the fast to fourteen hours or less, women can still experience the benefits that IF can have for weight loss and autophagy induction without putting themselves in any danger. This is not to say that women cannot fast in the same way that men can, but that they must start off slowly and gradually increase their hours of fasting so that they do not shock their bodies. When it comes to health, we must acknowledge the fact that the bodies of men and women are built differently and thus will respond differently to changes.

12 and 12

Women can also benefit from reducing their fasting window even further to 12 hours. This method can be beneficial in the beginning while your body gets used to the fasting, and you can gradually work your way up from here. In this method, you would normally only eat until three hours before you go to sleep, and then you could begin eating again early enough in the morning to have your first meal be breakfast. For example, if you go to bed at 10pm, you would only eat until 7pm. Then you could eat breakfast after 7am. This is beneficial for people who like to eat breakfast and who do not like to begin their day fasted.

For any person, regardless of their sex, the best approach to fasting may vary. When it comes to choosing an approach, being flexible is important. With dieting, the most important factor is consistency and so the best diet that you can choose for yourself will be the one that you can consistently maintain for a long enough period of time that your body can adjust, and changes can begin to occur.

Chapter 4. When To Avoid Intermittent Fasting

Although intermittent fasting is healthy, it is not a form of diet that we can all use. First and foremost, please speak to an advisor regarding intermittent fasting, particularly if you have identified medical problems before beginning your routine. If you're unclear whether intermittent fasting is appropriate for you, this list might point out explanations for maybe not doing it.

People with Eating Disorders

If you have an eating disorder or previously had an eating disorder, it could be safer to stop intermittent fasting. Anyone with eating disorders may have an obsessiveness with dieting, and it may be attributed to psychological factors and not anything that is physiologically wrong with you.

Diabetics

While intermittent fasting decreases insulin and can be helpful to those who avoid diabetes, in certain situations, it may not be a successful approach. If you do have diabetes, it's better to speak to the doctor because the variations in type 1 diabetes and type 2 diabetes in your particular case may mean that you don't have the correct intermittent fasting.

Serious Fitness Fanatics and Athletes

What if you're committed to a rigorous workout schedule already? Intermittent fasting will help you — and it can potentially hinder your success too. Athletes require calories, and their bodies are now functioning to lose fat and to strengthen their muscles. This intensity enables nutrition to be a huge factor in their success; through rest and good eating, they seek to cure their bodies, looking at their nutrients, not just calories. Athletes seem to use more calories, of course, than the normal individual who is not as active. Although intermittent fasting is achievable on a strict exercise schedule, proper planning is necessary to ensure that the body isn't overworking.

People Who Have Issues with Digestion

As if digestive problems were not too complicated to contend with on their own, introducing a wonky eating routine to the equation will just create further gastrointestinal discomfort. "If you have digestive issues (e.g., IBS), intermittent fasting can worsen the symptoms, or may even intensify digestive problems due to extended fasting bouts." Fasting cycles can interrupt the usual digestive system function, causing constipation, indigestion, and bloating. Gastrointestinal discomfort may be induced by consuming large meals – sometimes needed for IF forms that call for long-term fasting. "This is especially troubling for those with IBS who also have a more sensitive gut.

Nutrition, Concentration, and Motivation Are Critical to Everyday Activities

Food gives sustenance and strength that helps you to concentrate. When you're incredibly hungry, what you can think about is food that distracts the mind from the actual tasks at hand. If you have the sort of job or are involved in sports where strength and focus are required, intermittent fasting might not be appropriate for you.

Pregnant or Breastfeeding Women

Involving in it during pregnancy or breastfeeding may pose a risk to a child's health.

Pregnancy and breastfeeding need sufficient calorie consumption for the proper development of baby and milk productivity. Fasting cycles will mess with your food consumption, so breastfeeding and pregnant women shouldn't do intermittent fasting. "If you're attempting to get pregnant, IF may not be the diet of preference for you either. IF can even be related to fertility problems, triggering menstrual shifts, metabolic disturbances, and even early menopause in women.

People on Medications That Have to Be Taken with Food

These are several medicines that need to be consumed in the presence of food because without it, among many other side effects, they can render you feel nauseated or light-headed. Also, individuals who take a number of vitamins or nutrients per day may be impacted by IF fasting periods. For example, people who have a low blood iron count or anemia may need to take a daily iron supplement (or several) to help recover iron levels. Iron supplements are known for inducing diarrhea and can help alleviate the sensation when consuming it with meals. The moment you take an iron supplement can be adjustable, but what if you are on a medication that needs to be administered with food and at a very particular time of the day? That's where things get a bit messy because, in the end, getting into this diet is probably not a smart choice if it doesn't fit for the medications.

Those with A Weak Immune System or Have Cancer

Anyone that has undergone a significant illness previously, or are actually battling one, do not indulge in IF after first talking things up with a specialist. Here's why: "In most situations, sufficient calorie consumption is required to sustain lean body mass and a stable immune system that is vital for people with cancer or compromised immune systems," All people will speak to a specialist before trying intermittent fasting.

The Lifestyle Cannot Tolerate the Hours You Eat

Your job life will have a major effect on the willingness to participate in IF effectively. For instance, if you work the night shift and have to sleep in the afternoon because one of your feeding cycles comes in the afternoon, what do you do? Or worst, what if any of the fast happens when you are busy at work. Or, what if you work each day in various shifts and never have a regular schedule? Fasting cycles can trigger you to feel cold, with headaches and mood fluctuations. Having to deal with all those possible side effects could distract you from work and render you less efficient.

Chapter 5. Food To Eat and To Avoid During Intermittent Fasting

What To Eat

Berries

Berries are very healthy, incredibly flavorful, and much lower in calories and sugar than you might think! Their tart sweetness can really bring a smoothie to life, and they make an absolutely delicious snack on their own without any help from things like cream or sugar.

Cruciferous vegetables

These are the vegetables like cabbage, Brussels sprouts, broccoli, and cauliflower. These are wonderful additions to your diet because they're packed with vital nutrients and with fibre that your body will love and use with a quickness!

Eggs

Eggs are such a great addition to your diet because they're packed to the gills with Protein, you can do just about anything with them, they're easy to prepare, they travel well if you hard boil them, and they can pair with just about anything. They're a great Protein source for salads, and they're good on their own as well.

Fish

Fish are a wonderful source of Protein and healthy fats. White fish, in particular, is typically very lean, but fish like salmon that have a little bit of color in them are packed with Protein, fats, and oils that are great for you. They're good for brain and heart health, and there's a huge array of delicious things you can do with them.

Healthy starches like certain potatoes (with skins!)

Red potatoes, in particular, are perfectly fine to eat, even if you're trying to lose weight because your body can use those Carbs for fuel and the skins are packed with minerals that your body will enjoy. A little bit of potato here and there can-do good things for your nutrition, but they are also a great way to feel like you're getting a little more of those fun foods that you should cut back on.

Legumes

Beans, beans, the magical fruit. They're packed with Protein and the starch in them just makes them stick to your ribs without making you pay for it later. They're wonderful in soups, salads, and just about any other meal of the day that you're looking to fill out. By adding beans to your regimen, you might find that your meals stick with you a little bit longer and leave you feeling more satisfied than you thought possible.

Nuts

I know you've heard people talking about how a handful of almonds makes a great snack and if you're anything like me, you've always had kind of a hard time believing it. Nuts, as it turns out, have a good deal of their own healthy fats in them that your body can use to get through those rough patches and, while they are not the most satisfying snack on their own, you might consider topping your salad with them for a little bit of crunch, or pairing them with some berries to make them a little more satisfying.

Probiotics to help boost your gut health

Probiotics can be found in a number of different ways in health food stores, but they can make digestion and gut health much more optimum. Having a happy gut often means that your dietary success and overall health will improve!

Vegetables that are rich in healthy fats

Not to sound topical or trendy, but avocados are a great example of a vegetable that is packed with healthy fats. Look for vegetables with fatty acids and a higher fat content and you will find that if you add more of those into your regimen, you will get hungry less often.

Water, water, water, and more water

No matter what you decide to add to or subtract from your regimen, stay hydrated. This will aid in digestive health and ease, it will keep you from feeling as slumpy or tired, and it will keep you from getting too hungry. Add electrolytes where you need to and don't be shy about bringing a bottle with you when you go from place to place. Stay hydrated!

What To Avoid

Grains

While grains may have their health benefits and be full of fibre, you can also get these nutrients elsewhere. The human diet does not require grain consumption. The truth is while grains may have some benefits, they are ridiculously high in both total and net carbohydrates, making them incompatible with the ketogenic diet. A single serving of brown rice contains a shocking forty-two net Carbs, which is almost double your net Carbs intake for an entire day.

Although, some people do try what is known as the targeted ketogenic diet, which is a version of the diet specifically designed for those who complete extended and strenuous workouts. With the targeted ketogenic diet, a person will consume a small serving of a Carbs-heavy food, such as grains, thirty to forty minutes before working out.

Starchy Vegetables and Legumes

Some vegetables are high in carbohydrates. This includes potatoes, beans, beets, corn, and more. Yes, these vegetables may have nutritional benefits, but you can get these same nutrients in low-Carbs vegetable alternatives. To put into perspective how high in Carbs these options can be, a medium-sized white potato contains forty-three net Carbs (more than a serving of brown rice!), a standard sweet potato contains twenty-three net Carbs, and a serving of black beans contains twenty-five net Carbs.

Sugary Fruits

Most fruits contain a high sugar content, meaning that they are also high in carbohydrates, will spike your blood sugar, and cause an insulin reaction. To avoid this, it is important to avoid most fruits. The exception is that you can enjoy berries, lemons, and limes in moderation. Some people will also enjoy a small serving of melon as a treat from time to time, but watch your portion size as it can add up quickly!

Milk and Low-Fat Dairy Products

As you can enjoy dairy products such as cheese on the ketogenic diet, you may consider trying milk. Sadly, milk is much higher in carbohydrates than cheese, with a glass of two-percent milk containing twelve Carbs, half of your daily total. Instead, choose low-Carbs and dairy-free milk alternatives such as almond, coconut, and soy milk.

You may consider using low-fat cheeses instead of full fat to reduce the saturated fats you are consuming. But, if you are looking to reduce your saturated fat intake, choose lighter cuts of meat rather than low-fat dairy products. The reason for this is because when the cheese is made with low-fat dairy, it naturally has a higher carbohydrate content, which will cut into your daily net Carbs total.

Cashews, Pistachios, and Chestnuts

While you can enjoy nuts and seeds in moderation, keep in mind that nuts contain a moderate level of carbohydrates, and therefore should be eaten in moderation. However, some nuts are high in Carbs and thus are not fed on the ketogenic diet, including cashews, pistachios, and chestnuts.

If you want to enjoy nuts, instead of these options, you can fully enjoy almonds, pecans, walnuts, macadamia nuts, and other options.

Most Natural Sweeteners

While you can certainly enjoy sugar-free natural sweeteners such as stevia, monk fruit, and sugar alcohols, you should avoid natural sweeteners that contain sugar. Suffice to say the sugar content makes these sweeteners naturally high in Carbs. Not only that, but they will also spike your blood sugar and insulin. This means you should avoid things such as honey, agave, maple, coconut palm sugar, and dates.

Alcohol

Alcohol is not generally enjoyed on the ketogenic diet, as your body will be unable to burn off calories while your liver attempts to process alcohol. Many people also find that when they are in a state of ketosis, they get drunk more quickly and experience more severe hangovers. Not only that, but alcohol adds unnecessary calories and carbohydrates to your diet.

The worst offenders to choose would be margaritas, piña coladas, sangrias, Bloody Mary, whiskey sours, cosmopolitans, and regular beers.

But, if you do choose to drink alcohol regardless of drink in moderation and choose low-Carbs versions such as rum, vodka, tequila, whiskey, and gin. The next-best options would be dry wines and light beers.

Chapter 6. How To Start Intermittent Fasting

A lthough intermittent fasting is a very simple and straightforward approach yet, fasting can be an intimidating word for many. Our dependence on food for our physical, mental, and emotional satisfaction has increased to such an extent that even the thought of abstinence from food can make people anxious. This is even more important in the case of women as controlling hunger for them can be very difficult. Their mind is internally programmed to look for food consciously.

This is a reason that although intermittent fasting is very easy and simple, some people may find it difficult to follow it in the long run.

The main reason some people may find intermittent fasting difficult to follow is not due to the severity of hunger or their inability to manage their routine but because they have not followed proper procedures.

Yes, you have read it right! The biggest reason people are unable to follow intermittent fasting is that they don't follow the process properly. They are so enthusiastic about losing weight that they don't give time to their bodies to prepare for the fasting schedules.

You must understand that humans have also evolved from animal species. Our first and foremost instinct is and always would be to eat, sleep, and procreate. If any obstruction is put in the way of either of these things, the initial reaction of our body would be adverse. If you try to snatch away any of these things or enforce stricter rules in these areas, the results are not going to be favorable.

No matter how beneficial fasting is for the body, the body is not going to react well to it initially. You will face the hunger pangs, cramps, distraction, mind wandering around food, irritability, and mood swings. There are ways to manage all these symptoms, but there can be no denying the fact that these issues will arise.

You can lower these adverse reactions by following proper protocols, and intermittent fasting will become a life-changing experience for you. If you jump the steps and rush to the last part in the first leg, you are bound to have severe symptoms, and not only the results would get affected, but you will also face problems in managing the lifestyle for long.

A Step-by-Step Approach

The best way to approach intermittent fasting is to move step by step. You must never undermine the fact that our lifestyles are heavily centered around food. There are shorter gaps between meals. There is a high amount of Carbs-intake that also aggravates the situation to a great extent.

If you follow a very hard approach from the word GO, you are bound to face adjustment issues. The best approach is to allow the body to adapt to the fasting schedule and let it build the capacity to stay hungry.

Eliminate Snacks

This is something that would come several times in this book. It is a very important thing that you must understand. The root cause of most of our health issues is the habit of frequent snacking.

Snacking leads to 2 major issues:

It keeps causing repeated glucose spikes that invoke an insulin response and hence the overall insulin presence in the bloodstream increases aggravating the problem of insulin resistance.

It usually involves refined Carbs and sugar-rich food items that will lead to cravings, and you will keep feeling the urge to eat at even shorter intervals.

This is a reason your preparation for intermittent fasting must begin with the elimination of snacks. You can have 2-3 nutrient-dense meals in a day, but you will have to remove the habit of snacking from your routine.

As long as the habit of snacking is there, you'll have a very hard time staying away from food as this habit never allows your ghrelin response clock to get set at fixed intervals. This means that you will keep having urges to eat sweets and Carbs-rich foods, and you will also have strong hunger pangs at regular intervals.

The solution to this problem is very simple. You can take 2-3 nutrient-dense meals that are rich in fat, Protein, and fibre. Such a meal will not only provide you with adequate energy for the day but would also keep your gut engaged for long so that you don't have frequent hunger pangs.

The farther you can stay away from refined Carbs-rich and sugar-rich food items, the easier you would find it to deal with hunger.

You must start easy. Don't do anything drastic or earth-shattering.

Simply start by lowering the number of snacks you have in a day. The snacks have not only become a need of the body, but they are also a part of the habit. In a day, there are numerous instances when we eat titbits that we don't care about. We sip cold-drinks, sweetened beverages, chips, cookies, bagels, donuts, burgers, pizzas simply because they are in front of us or accessible. We have made food an excuse to take breaks. This habit will have to be broken if you want to move on the path of good health.

Widen the Gap Between Your Meals

This is the second step in your preparation. You must start widening the gap between your meals. This process needs to be gradual and should only begin when you have eliminated snacks from your routine. Two nutrient-dense meals in a day or two meals and a smaller meal or lunch comprising of fibre-rich salads should be your goal.

However, you must remember that these two steps must be taken over a long period. You must allow your body to get used to the change. There would be a temptation that it is easy to follow these, and you can jump to the actual intermittent fasting routine, but it is very important to avoid all such temptations as they are only going to lead to failures.

If your body doesn't get used to this routine, very soon, you'll start feeling trapped. You'll start finding ways to cheat the routine. You'll look for excuses to violate the routine, and it very soon becomes a habit. This is the reason you must allow your body to take some time to adjust to the new schedule.

You should remember that intermittent fasting is a way of life. This might slower the results, but it is going to make your overall journey smoother and better.

Example of Food Plan

Following a meal plan is highly essential if you want to lose weight. When you combine your meal plans with intermittent fasting, you will begin to see massive results. Women above 50 need to keep track of their meals as they face the reality of gaining weight easier than losing it.

Days	Breakfast	Snack	Lunch	Snack	Dinner
Monday	One large grapefruit and 3 Scrambled Eggs	25 almonds	One apple Turkey Wrap	A piece of string cheese	Spicy Chicken with Side salad, dressing with two tablespoons of olive oil or vinegar
Tuesday	One large grapefruit, ham, and Lean Eggs	25 almonds	One apple, Cheese Burrito, and Black Bean	A piece of string cheese	Bun and Veggie Burger together with a salad dressed with four tablespoons of olive oil or vinegar, and finally one serving of sweet potato fries
Wednesday	Zero-fat Greek yogurt and Berry Wafflewich	Two tablespoons of hummus and 15 snap peas	One apple and Gobbleguac Sandwich	One piece of string cheese and banana	Two cups of broccoli, One cup of brown rice, and Steamed Snapper together with Pesto
Thursday	One large grapefruit and zero-fat Greek yogurt	One Luna Bar	25 almonds and the I-Am-Not-Eating-Salad Salad	Four tablespoons of hummus and 30 baby carrots	Two cups of snow peas, a cup of brown rice and Chicken Spinach Parmesan

Friday	One banana and Loaded Vegetable Omelet	One piece of string cheese	One apple and a Turkey Wrap	Two tablespoons of hummus and ten cherry tomatoes	Two cups of broccoli, rice with Quick Lemon Chicken
Saturday	One large grapefruit and three Scrambled Eggs	25 almonds	Leftover cups of broccoli, Chicken Marengo and Penne	Zero-fat Greek yogurt and piece of string cheese	Two cups of snow peas and Thai Beef Lettuce Wraps
Sunday	One banana and Loaded Vegetable Omelet	Zero-fat Greek yogurt and piece of string cheese	One apple and the I-Am-Not-Eating-Salad Salad	One Luna Bar and teen cherry tomatoes	One cup of brown rice, 2 cups of broccoli and Tofu Stir-Fry

Chapter 7. Breakfast Recipes

1. Seed and Nut Bread

Preparation time: 10 minutes
Cooking time: 40 minutes
Servings: 12
Ingredients:
- 3 eggs
- ¼ cup avocado oil
- 1 tsp. psyllium husk powder
- 1 tsp. apple cider vinegar
- ¾ tsp. salt
- 5 drops liquid stevia
- 1 ½ cups raw unsalted almonds
- ½ cup raw unsalted pepitas
- ½ cup raw unsalted sunflower seeds
- ½ cup flaxseeds

Directions:
1. Preheat the oven to 325°F. Line a loaf pan with parchment paper.
2. In a huge bowl, whisk together the oil, eggs, psyllium husk powder, vinegar, salt, and liquid stevia.
3. Stir in the pepitas, almonds, sunflower seeds, and flaxseeds until well combined.
4. Pour the batter into the prepared loaf pan, smooth it out and let it rest for 2 minutes.
5. Bake for 40 minutes.
6. Cool, slice, and serve.

Nutrition: Calories: 131 - Fat: 12g - Carbs: 4g - Protein: 5g.

2. Chia Breakfast Bowl

Preparation time: 10 minutes
Cooking time: 0 minutes
Servings: 2
Ingredients:
- ¼ cup whole chia seeds
- 2 cups almond milk, unsweetened
- 2 tbsp. sugar-free maple syrup
- 1 tsp. vanilla extract

Toppings:
- Cinnamon and extra maple syrup
- Nuts and berries

Directions:
1. Combine the syrup, milk, chia seeds, and vanilla extract in a bowl and stir to mix.
2. Let stand for 30 minutes, then whisk.
3. Transfer to an airtight container.
4. Cover and refrigerate overnight.
5. Serve in the morning.

Nutrition: Calories: 298 - Fat: 15g - Carbs: 5g - Protein: 14g.

3. Ricotta Omelet with Swiss Chard

Preparation time: 10 minutes
Cooking time: 15 minutes
Servings: 2
Ingredients:
- 6 eggs
- 2 tbsp. almond milk
- ½ tsp. kosher salt
- ½ tsp. ground black pepper
- 6 tbsp. unsalted butter, divided
- 2 bunch Swiss chard, cleaned and stemmed
- 2/3 cup ricotta

Directions:
1. Add the eggs, and milk. Season with salt and pepper then whisk. Set aside.
2. In a skillet, melt 4 tbsp. butter. Add the veggie leaves and sauté until just wilted. Remove from pan. Set aside.
3. Now melt 1 tbsp. butter in the skillet.
4. Add half of the egg mixture. Spread the mixture. Cook for about 2 minutes.
5. Add half of the ricotta when the edges are firm, but the center is still a bit runny.
6. Bend 1/3 of the omelet over the ricotta filling. Transfer to a plate.
7. Repeat with the remaining butter and egg mixture.
8. Serve with Swiss chard.

Nutrition: Calories: 693 - Fat: 60g - Carbs: 8g - Protein: 2g.

4. Omelet with Goat Cheese and Herb

Preparation time: 5 minutes
Cooking time: 12 minutes
Servings: 2
Ingredients:

- 6 eggs, beaten
- 2 tbsp. chopped herbs (basil, parsley or cilantro)
- Kosher salt and black pepper to taste
- 2 tbsp. unsalted butter
- 4oz. fresh goat cheese

Directions:

1. Whisk together the eggs, herbs, salt, and pepper.
2. Melt 1 tbsp. butter in a skillet.
3. Put half of the egg mixture and cook for 4 to 5 minutes, or until just set.
4. Crumble half the goat cheese over the eggs and fold in half.
5. Cook for 1 minute, or until cheese is melted. Transfer to a plate.
6. Repeat process with the remaining butter, egg mixture, and goat cheese.
7. Serve.

Nutrition: Calories: 523 - Fat: 43g - Carbs: 3g - Protein: 31g.

5. Bacon and Zucchini Egg Breakfast

Preparation time: 10 minutes
Cooking time: 10 minutes
Servings: 2
Ingredients:

- 2 cups zucchini noodles
- 2 slices of raw bacon
- ¼ cup grated Asiago cheese
- 2 eggs
- Salt and pepper to taste

Directions:

1. Cut the bacon slices into ¼ inch thick strips.
2. Cook the bacon in a pan for 3 minutes.
3. Add the zucchini and mix well.
4. Season with salt and pepper.
5. Flatten slightly with a spatula and make 2 depressions for the eggs.
6. Sprinkle with the cheese.
7. Break one egg into each dent.
8. Cook 3 minutes more, then cover and cook for 2 to 4 minutes, or until the eggs are cooked.
9. Serve.

Nutrition: Calories: 242 - Fat: 19g - Carbs: 4g - Protein: 14g.

6. Cinnamon Roll Oatmeal

Preparation time: 10 minutes
Cooking time: 10 minutes
Servings: 2
Ingredients:

- 1/3 cup crushed pecans
- 1 tbsp. flaxseed meal
- 1 tbsp. chia seeds
- 2 tbsp. cauliflower, riced
- 1 cup plus 1 tbsp. coconut milk
- 1 tbsp. heavy cream
- 1 oz. cream cheese
- 1 tbsp. butter
- ½ tsp. cinnamon
- ½ tsp. maple flavor
- ¼ tsp. vanilla essence
- Pinch of nutmeg
- Pinch of allspice
- 1 tbsp. erythritol, powdered
- 5 drops liquid stevia
- Pinch of xanthan gum

Directions:

1. In a bowl, add flax seeds and chia seeds and set aside.
2. Heat the coconut milk in a saucepan. Once warm, add the cauliflower and cook until it starts to boil.
3. Lower the heat and add allspice, nutmeg, vanilla, maple flavor, and cinnamon.
4. Add stevia and erythritol to the pan and stir well.
5. Add the chia seed and flaxseed mixture to the pan and mix well.
6. Once the mixture is hot, add the cream, cream cheese, butter, and pecans.
7. Mix well and serve.

Nutrition: Calories: 398 - Fat: 37.8g - Carbs: 3.1g Protein: 8.8g.

7. Turkey and Scrambled Eggs Breakfast

Preparation time: 10 minutes
Cooking time: 15 minutes
Servings: 2
Ingredients:

- 4 slices avocado
- Salt and pepper to taste
- 4 slices bacon, diced
- 4 turkey breast slices, cooked
- 4 tbsp. coconut oil
- 4 eggs, whisked

Directions:

1. Heat a pan over medium heat.
2. Add bacon slices and brown all over.
3. Heat oil in another pan.
4. Add eggs, salt, and pepper, and scramble.
5. Divide turkey breast slices, bacon, scrambled eggs, and avocado slices on 2 plates and serve.

Nutrition: Calories: 791- Fat: 64.3g - Carbs: 8.8g Protein: 41.8g.

8. Breakfast Cereal

Preparation time: 5 minutes
Cooking time: 3 minutes
Servings: 2
Ingredients:

- ½ cup shredded coconut, unsweetened
- 4 tsp. butter
- 2 cups almond milk, unsweetened
- 1 tbsp. stevia
- Pinch of salt
- 2 tbsp. macadamia nuts, chopped
- 2 tbsp. walnuts, chopped
- 1/3 cup flaxseed

Directions:

1. Melt the butter in a pan.
2. Add the coconut, milk, salt, nuts, flaxseed, and stevia, and stir well.
3. Cook for 3 minutes and stir again.
4. Remove from heat. Set aside for 10 minutes.
5. Serve.

Nutrition: Calories: 588 - Fat: 48g - Carbs: 6.8g Protein: 16.5g.

9. Best Intermittent Bread

Preparation time: 10 minutes
Cooking time: 30 minutes
Servings: 8
Ingredients:

- 1 ½ cup almond flour
- 6 drops liquid stevia
- 1 pinch Pink Himalayan salt
- ¼ tsp. cream of tartar
- 3 tsp. baking powder
- ¼ cup butter, melted
- 6 large eggs, separated

Directions:

1. Preheat the oven to 375°F.
2. To the egg whites, add cream of tartar and beat until soft peaks are formed.
3. In a food processor, combine stevia, salt, baking powder, almond flour, melted butter, 1/3 of the beaten egg whites, and egg yolks. Mix well.
4. Then add the remaining 2/3 of the egg whites and gently process until fully mixed. Don't over mix.
5. Put a grease on a (8 x 4) loaf pan and pour the mixture in it.
6. Bake for 30 minutes.
7. Enjoy.

Nutrition: Calories: 90 - Fat: 7g - Carbs: 2g Protein: 3g.

10.   Bread De Soul

Preparation time: 10 minutes
Cooking time: 45 minutes
Servings: 16
Ingredients:

- ¼ tsp. cream of tartar
- 2 ½ tsp. baking powder
- 1 tsp. xanthan gum
- 1/3 tsp. baking soda
- ½ tsp. salt
- 2/3 cup unflavored whey Protein
- ¼ cup olive oil
- ¼ cup heavy whipping cream
- Drops of sweet leaf stevia
- 4 eggs
- ¼ cup butter
- 12oz. softened cream cheese

Directions:

1. Preheat the oven to 325°F.
2. In a bowl, microwave cream cheese and butter for 1 minute.
3. Remove and blend well with a hand mixer.
4. Add olive oil, eggs, heavy cream, and few drops of sweetener and blend well.
5. Put together the dry ingredients in a separate bowl.
6. Combine the dry ingredients with the wet ingredients and mix with a spoon. Don't use a hand blender to avoid whipping it too much.
7. Grease a bread pan and pour the mixture into the pan.
8. Bake in the oven until golden brown for about 45 minutes.
9. Cool and serve.

Nutrition: Calories: 200 - Fat: 15.2g - Carbs: 1.8g Protein: 10g.

11.   Chia Seed Bread

Preparation time: 10 minutes
Cooking time: 4 minutes
Servings: 16
Ingredients:

- ½ tsp. xanthan gum
- ½ cup butter
- 2 Tbsp. coconut oil
- Tbsp. baking powder
- Tbsp. sesame seeds
- Tbsp. chia seeds
- ½ tsp. salt
- ¼ cup sunflower seeds
- 2 cups almond flour
- 7 eggs

Directions:

1. Preheat the oven to 350°F.
2. Beat eggs in a bowl for 1 to 2 minutes.
3. Beat in the xanthan gum and combine coconut oil and melted butter into eggs, beating continuously.
4. Set aside the sesame seeds, but add the rest of the ingredients.
5. Get a loaf pan with baking paper and place the mixture in it. Top the mixture with sesame seeds.
6. Bake in the oven for about 35 to 40 minutes.

Nutrition: Calories: 405 - Fat: 37g - Carbs: 4g Protein: 14g.

12.   Special Intermittent Bread

Preparation time: 15 minutes
Cooking time: 40 minutes
Servings: 14
Ingredients:
- 2 tsp. baking powder
- ½ cup water
- 1 tbsp. poppy seeds
- 2 cups fine ground almond meal
- 5 large eggs
- ½ cup olive oil
- ½ tsp. fine Himalayan salt

Directions:
1. Preheat oven to 400°F.
2. In a bowl, combine salt, almond meal, and baking powder.
3. Drip in oil while mixing, until it forms a crumbly dough.
4. Make a little round hole in the middle of the dough and pour eggs into the middle of the dough.
5. Pour water and whisk eggs together with the mixer in the small circle until it is frothy.
6. Start making larger circles to combine the almond meal mixture with the dough until you have a smooth and thick batter.
7. Line your loaf pan with parchment paper.
8. Pour batter into the loaf pan and sprinkle poppy seeds on top.
9. Bake in the oven for 40 minutes in the center rack until firm and golden brown.
10. Cool in the oven for 30 minutes.
11. Slice and serve.

Nutrition: Calories: 227 - Fat: 21g - Carbs: 4g Protein: 7g.

13.   Intermittent Fluffy Cloud Bread

Preparation time: 25 minutes
Cooking time: 25 minutes
Servings: 3
Ingredients:
- Pinch salt
- ½ tbsp. ground psyllium husk powder
- ½ tbsp. baking powder
- ¼ tsp. cream of tarter
- 3 eggs, separated
- ½ cup, cream cheese

Directions:
1. Preheat oven to 300°F.
2. Whisk egg whites in a bowl until soft peaks are formed.
3. Mix egg yolks with cream cheese, salt, cream of tartar, psyllium husk powder, and baking powder in a bowl.
4. Fold in the egg whites carefully and transfer to the baking tray.
5. Place in the oven and bake for 25 minutes.
6. Remove from the oven and serve.

Nutrition: Calories: 185 - Fat: 16.4g - Carbs: 3.9g Protein: 6.6g.

14.   Puri Bread

Preparation time: 10 minutes
Cooking time: 5 minutes
Servings: 6
Ingredients:
- 1 cup almond flour, sifted
- ½ cup of warm water
- 1 tbsp clarified butter
- 1 cup olive oil for frying
- Salt to taste

Directions:
1. Salt the water and add the flour.
2. Create a hole in the center of the dough and pour warm clarified butter.
3. Knead the dough and let stand for 15 minutes, covered.
4. Shape into 6 balls.
5. Flatten the balls into 6 thin rounds using a rolling pin.
6. Heat enough oil to cover a round frying pan completely.
7. Place a puri in it when hot.
8. Fry for 20 seconds on each side.
9. Place on a paper towel.
10. Repeat with the rest of the puri and serve.

Nutrition: Calories: 106 - Fat: 3g - Carbs: 6g - Protein: 3g.

15. Intermittent Bakers Bread

Preparation time: 10 minutes
Cooking time: 20 minutes
Servings: 12
Ingredients:

- Pinch of salt
- 4 tbsp. light cream cheese; softened
- ½ tsp. cream of tartar
- 4 eggs, yolks, and whites separated

Directions:

1. Heat 2 racks in the middle of the oven at 350°F.
2. Line 2 baking pan with parchment paper, then grease with cooking spray.
3. Separate egg yolks from the whites. Put in separate mixing bowls.
4. Beat the egg whites and cream of tartar with a hand mixer until stiff, about 3 to 5 minutes. Do not over-beat.
5. Whisk the cream cheese, salt, and egg yolks until smooth.
6. Slowly fold the cheese mix into the whites until fluffy.
7. Spoon ¼ cup measure of the batter onto the baking sheets, 6 mounds on each sheet.
8. Bake for 20 to 22 minutes, alternating racks halfway through.
9. Cool and serve.

Nutrition: Calories: 41- Fat: 3.2g - Carbs: 1g Protein: 2.4g.

16. Cheese Garlic Bread

Preparation time: 10 minutes
Cooking time: 15 minutes
Servings: 10
Ingredients:

- 6oz. mozzarella cheese; shredded
- 3oz. almond meal
- 1 tbsp. crushed garlic
- 1 tbsp. full fat cream cheese
- 1 tsp. baking powder
- 1 tbsp. dried parsley
- 1 medium egg
- 1 pinch salt

Directions:

1. Add every ingredient into a bowl, excluding the egg.
2. Lightly stir the mixture until combined.
3. Place bowl in a microwave and microwave for 1 minute on high.
4. Stir mixture and microwave for 30 seconds more.
5. Add the egg into the dough and gently stir until incorporated.
6. Add mixture onto a prepared baking tray and mold into a loaf shape.
7. Sprinkle any leftover cheese over the bread.
8. Bake loaf for 15 minutes at 425F, or until golden brown.

Nutrition: Calories: 117.4 - Fat: 9.8g Carbs: 2.4g - Protein: 6.2g.

17. Avocado Salad Dish

Preparation time: 8 minutes
Cooking time: 5 minutes
Servings: 2
Ingredients:

- ½ of a medium avocado, sliced
- 1 tbsp apple cider vinegar
- 1 tbsp olive oil
- 4oz. chopped lettuce
- 4 slices of bacon, chopped

Directions:

1. Prepare bacon and for this, put a skillet pan over medium heat and when hot, put chopped bacon and let it cook for 5 to 8 minutes until golden brown.
2. Then distribute lettuce and avocado between two plates, top with bacon, drizzle with olive oil and apple cider and serve.

Nutrition: Calories:14 - Fat: 6g - Protein: 2g - Carbs: 1g.

18. Sausage Styled Rolled Omelet

Preparation time: 5 minutes
Cooking time: 8 minutes
Servings: 2
Ingredients:

- 1 tbsp chopped spinach
- 1 tbsp whipped topping
- 2 eggs
- 2oz. ground turkey
- 1 tbsp grated mozzarella cheese

Directions:

1. Bring out a skillet pan, put it over medium heat, add ground turkey and cook for 5 minutes until cooked through.
2. Meanwhile, crack eggs in a bowl, add whipped topping and spinach and whisk until combined.
3. When the meat is cooked, put it to a plate, then switch heat to the low level and pour in the egg mixture.
4. Cook the eggs for 3 minutes until the bottom is firm, then flip it and cook for 3 minutes until the omelet is firmed, covering the pan.
5. Sprinkle cheese on the omelet, cook for 1 minute until cheese has melted, and then slide omelet to a plate.
6. Spread ground meat on the omelet, roll it, then cut it in half and serve.

Nutrition: Calories: 126 - Fat: 9g - Protein: 10g - Carbs: 1g.

19. Almond Flour Lemon Bread

Preparation time: 15 minutes
Cooking time: 45 minutes
Servings: 2
Ingredients:

- 1 tsp. French herbs
- 2 tsp. lemon juice
- 1 tsp. salt
- 1 tsp. cream of tartar
- 2 tsp. baking powder
- ¼ cup melted butter
- 5 large eggs, divided
- ¼ cup coconut flour
- 1 ½ cup almond flour

Directions:

1. Preheat the oven to 350°F. Beat the whites and cream of tartar until soft peaks form.
2. In a bowl, combine salt, egg yolks, melted butter, and lemon juice. Mix well.
3. Add coconut flour, almond flour, herbs, and baking powder. Mix well.
4. To the dough, add 1/3 the egg whites and mix until well-combined.
5. Add the remaining egg whites mixture and slowly mix to incorporate everything. Do not over mix.
6. Put a grease on a loaf pan with butter or coconut oil.
7. Pour mixture into the loaf pan and bake for 30 minutes.

Nutrition: Calories: 115 - Fat: 9.9g - Carbs: 3.3g Protein: 5.2g.

20. Buttermilk Pancakes

Preparation time: 5 minutes
Cooking time: 8 minutes
Servings: 2
Ingredients:

- 1 ½ tbsp. coconut flour
- 1 ½ tbsp. almond flour
- 1 egg
- 2 tbsp. almond milk + ¼ tsp. apple cider vinegar, mixed in a bowl
- ¼ tsp. vanilla extract
- Pinch of baking powder
- ½ tsp. erythritol
- 1 tsp. butter, melted
- Pinch of sea salt

Directions:

1. Mix all the ingredients in a bowl.
2. Heat a lightly greased skillet over medium-high heat. Make sure the skillet is hot.
3. Spoon batter onto the skillet and cook until the batter starts to bubble, about 2 minutes. Then flip and cook until middle is done. Adjust the heat if needed.
4. Repeat with the remaining batter.
5. Serve with condiments of choice.

Nutrition: Calories: 81- Fat: 6g - Carbs: 4g - Protein: 3g.

21. Power Cream with Strawberry

Preparation time: 5 minutes
Cooking time: 0
Servings: 2
Ingredients:
- 1 tbsp coconut oil
- 1 tsp vanilla extract, unsweetened
- 2oz. coconut cream, full-fat
- 2oz. fresh strawberries

Directions:
1. Bring out a large bowl, put all the ingredients in it and then mix by using a blender until smooth.
2. Distribute evenly between two bowls and then serve.

Nutrition: Calories:214 - Fat: 3g - Protein: 4g - Carbs: 2g.

22. Savory Intermittent Pancake

Preparation time: 5 minutes
Cooking time: 5 minutes
Servings: 2
Ingredients:
- ¼ cup almond flour
- ½ tbsp unsalted butter
- 2 eggs
- 1oz. cream cheese, softened

Directions:
1. Bring out a bowl, crack eggs in it, whisk well until fluffy, and then whisk in flour and cream cheese until well combined.
2. Bring out a skillet pan, put it over medium heat, add butter and when it melts, drop pancake batter in four sections, spread it evenly, and cook for 2 minutes per side until brown.

Nutrition: Calories: 167 - Fat: 15g - Protein: 2g - Carbs: 1g.

23. Mix Veggie Fritters

Preparation time: 5 minutes
Cooking time: 7 minutes
Servings: 2
Ingredients:
- ½ tsp nutritional yeast
- 1oz. chopped broccoli
- 2oz. zucchini, grated, squeezed
- 2 eggs
- 4 tbsp almond flour

Directions:
1. Wrap grated zucchini in a cheesecloth, twist it well to remove excess moisture, and then Put zucchini in a bowl.
2. Add remaining ingredients, except for oil, and then whisk well until combined.
3. Bring out a skillet pan, put it over medium heat, add oil and when hot, drop zucchini mixture in four portions, shape them into flat patties and cook for 4 minutes per side until thoroughly cooked.

Nutrition: Calories: 191 - Fat: 10g - Protein: 1g - Carbs: 1g.

24. Spinach and Eggs Mix

Preparation time: 5 minutes
Cooking time: 20 minutes
Servings: 4
Ingredients:
- 2 tablespoons olive oil
- ½ teaspoon smoked paprika
- 8 eggs, whisked
- 2 cups baby spinach
- Salt and black pepper to the taste

Directions:
1. Combine all ingredients in a bowl except the oil and whisk them well.
2. Heat up your air fryer at 360°F, add the oil, heat it up, add the eggs and spinach mix, cover, cook for 20 minutes, divide between plates and serve.

Nutrition: Calories: 220 - Fat: 11g - Fibre: 3g - Carbs: 4g -Protein: 6g.

25. Savory Ham and Cheese Waffles

Preparation Time: 10 minutes
Cooking Time: 10 minutes
Servings: 2
Ingredients:
- 2oz. ham steak, chopped
- 2oz. cheddar cheese, grated
- 6 eggs
- 1 teaspoon baking powder
- Basil, to taste
- 12 tablespoons butter, melted
- Olive oil, as needed
- 1-teaspoon sea salt

Special Equipment:
- A waffle iron

Directions:
1. Preheat the waffle iron and set aside.
2. Crack the eggs and keep the egg yolks and egg whites in two separate bowls.
3. Add the butter, baking powder, basil, and salt to the egg yolks. Whisk well. Fold in the chopped ham and stir until well combined. Set aside.
4. Lightly season the egg whites with salt and beat until it forms stiff peaks.
5. Add the egg whites into the bowl of egg yolk mixture. Allow to sit for about 5 minutes.
6. Lightly coat the waffle iron with the olive oil. Slowly pour half of the mixture in the waffle iron and cook for about 4 minutes. Repeat with the remaining egg mixture.
7. Take off from the waffle iron and serve warm on two serving plates.

Nutrition: Calories: 636 - Fat: 50.2g - Carbs: 1.1g Protein: 45.1g.

26. Classic Spanakopita Frittata

Preparation Time: 10 minutes
Cooking Time: 3-4 hours
Servings: 8
Ingredients:
- 12 eggs, beaten
- ½ cup feta cheese
- 1 cup heavy whipping cream
- 2 cups spinach, chopped
- 2 teaspoons garlic, minced
- 2 tablespoons extra-virgin olive oil

Directions:
1. Grease the bottom of the slow cooker, put with the olive oil lightly.
2. Stir together the beaten eggs, feta cheese, heavy cream, spinach, and garlic until well combined.
3. Slowly pour the mixture into the slow cooker. Cook covered on LOW for 3 to 4 hours, or until a knife inserted in the center comes out clean.
4. Take off from the slow cooker and cool for about 3 minutes before slicing.

Nutrition: Calories: 254 - Fat: 22.3g - Fibre: 0g - Carbs: 2.1g - Protein: 11.1g - Cholesterol: 364mg.

27.   Intermittent Tacos with Guacamole and Bacon

Preparation Time: 5 minutes
Cooking Time: 10 minutes
Servings: 2
Ingredients:

- 1/4 cup organic romaine lettuce (chopped)
- 3 tablespoons organic sweet potatoes (diced and cooked)
- 1 tablespoon Brain Octane Oil
- 1 tablespoon ghee (grass-fed)
- 2 eggs (pasture-raised)
- 1 medium avocado (organic)
- 3 slices pastured bacon (cooked)
- 1/4 teaspoon Himalayan pink salt
- Organic micro cilantro (for garnish)

Directions:

1. In a skillet over medium heat, heat up the ghee.
2. Get an egg. Crack the egg in the middle of the skillet. Poke the egg yolk.
3. Let the egg cook until solid for about 2 minutes per side. Transfer the cooked egg onto a plate lined with paper towels to absorb the excess oil.
4. Cook the other egg in a similar way. The 2 cooked eggs will serve as the taco shells.
5. In a mixing bowl, put in the avocado, pink salt, and octane oil. Mash the avocado and mix well.
6. Equally divide the avocado mixture into 2 portions. Spread each avocado mixture onto each egg taco.
7. Arrange the romaine lettuce on top of each taco shell.
8. Put a bacon slice on each taco. Top each taco with the cooked sweet potatoes.
9. Garnish the tacos with micro cilantro and sprinkle some pink salt for added taste.
10. Fold each taco in half. Serve.

Nutrition: Calories: 387 - Carbs: 9g - Fat: 35g - Protein: 11g – Fibre: 5g.

28.   Sausage Stuffed Bell Peppers

Preparation Time: 15 minutes
Cooking Time: 4-5 hours
Servings: 4
Ingredients:

- 1 cup breakfast sausage, crumbled
- 4 bell peppers, seedless and cut the top
- ½ cup coconut milk
- 6 eggs
- 1 cup cheddar cheese, shredded
- 1 tablespoon extra-virgin olive oil
- ½ teaspoon freshly ground black pepper

Directions:

1. Add the coconut milk, eggs, and black pepper in a medium bowl, whisking until smooth. Set aside.
2. Line your slow cooker insert with aluminum foil. Grease the aluminum foil with 1 tablespoon olive oil.
3. Evenly stuff four bell peppers with the crumbled sausage, and spoon the egg mixture into the peppers.
4. Arrange the stuffed peppers in the slow cooker. Sprinkle the cheese on top.
5. Cook covered on low for 4 or 5 hours, or until the peppers are browned and the eggs are completely set.
6. Divide in 4 serving plates and serve warm.

Nutrition: Calories: 459 - Fat: 36.3g - Protein: 25.2g - Carbs: 7.9g - Fibre: 3g - Cholesterol: 376mg.

29.   Zucchini Pancakes

Preparation Time: 5 minutes
Cooking Time: 10 minutes
Servings: 3
Ingredients:

- 1,5 oz. zucchini
- ½ cup almond flour
- 2 tbsp. coconut flour
- 2oz. full-fat milk
- 3 eggs
- ½ tsp baking powder
- 1 tsp cinnamon
- 1 tbsp. ghee butter
- Salt and erythritol to taste

Directions:

1. Grate the zucchini, season with salt and place into a sieve to drain
2. Put into a blender, add other ingredients, pulse well
3. Heat then melt the butter in a pan in medium heat
4. Form the pancakes and put into the skillet
5. Close the lid and cook 3 minutes each side

Nutrition: Calories: 130 - Carbs: 0,7g - Fat: 7g - Protein: 7,5g.

30.   Shrimp Omelet

Preparation Time: 5 minutes
Cooking Time: 15 minutes
Servings: 4
Ingredients:

- 10oz. boiled shrimps
- 10 eggs
- 4 tbsp. ghee butter
- 4 garlic cloves
- 1 cup intermittent mayo
- 1 fresh red chilli peppers
- 1 tbsp. olive oil
- 1 tsp cumin powder

Directions:

1. Mince the garlic cloves and chilli pepper
2. In a bowl, blend the shrimps with the mayo, olive oil, minced chilli pepper, cumin, minced garlic, salt, and pepper. Set aside for a while
3. In the other bowl, whisk the eggs then add salt and pepper
4. Heat the ghee butter in the skillet, add eggs and shrimp mixture
5. Cook for 5-6 minutes, serve hot

Nutrition: Calories: 855 - Carbs: 4g - Fat: 82g - Protein: 27g.

31.   Cauliflower Patties

Preparation Time: 11 minutes
Cooking Time: 15 minutes
Servings: 2
Ingredients:

- 10oz. cauliflower
- 1 tbsp. yeast
- 2/3 cup almond flour
- ½ tsp cumin powder
- ½ tsp paprika
- 2 eggs
- 1 tbsp. ghee butter
- Salt and pepper to taste

Directions:

1. Divide the cauliflower into florets, put them in a pot and boil for 8-10 min
2. Remove to a plate and let it rest for 3-4 min
3. Meanwhile, in a bowl combine the eggs, paprika, cumin, yeast, pepper, salt
4. Put the cauliflower in a blender and pulse till even
5. Add the cauliflower to the bowl with other mixed ingredients, mix well and form the patties
6. Heat the ghee butter in a skillet over medium heat, cook the patties for 3-5 min per side

Nutrition: Calories: 235 - Carbs: 5g - Fat: 23g - Protein: 6g.

32.   Spinach Sandwich

Preparation Time: 7 minutes
Cooking Time: 8 minutes
Servings: 1
Ingredients:
- ½ avocado
- 2oz. spinach
- 2oz. cheddar cheese
- 1 tbsp. coconut oil
- 2 cherry tomatoes
- Salt and pepper to taste

Directions:
1. Mince the spinach; place it in a small plate. Make a round cutlet out of it
2. Grate the cheese, slice the avocado and cut tomatoes in halves
3. Sprinkle the oil on the leaves, place the grated cheddar cheese, avocado, and tomato on top of it. Season with salt and pepper

Nutrition: Calories: 419 - Carbs: 4g - Fat: 43g - Protein: 4g.

33.   Fried Eggs with Bacon

Preparation Time: 5 minutes
Cooking Time: 10 minutes
Servings: 4
Ingredients:
- 8 medium eggs
- 5oz. bacon
- 2 medium tomatoes
- 1 tsp chopped parsley
- 1 tbsp. ghee butter
- Salt to taste

Directions:
1. Heat the ghee butter in a skillet over medium-high heat

2. Slice the bacon and fry it until crispy for 3-4 minutes, then set aside on a paper towel
3. Meanwhile, cut the tomatoes in small cubes
4. Crack the eggs in the same skillet, add tomatoes, season with salt and cook till the desired readiness
5. Top with the bacon and parsley. Serve hot

Nutrition: Calories: 273 - Carbs: 1g - Fat: 22g - Protein: 15g.

34.   Classic Steak 'n Eggs

Preparation Time: 5 minutes
Cooking Time: 15 minutes
Servings: 4
Ingredients:
- 8 eggs
- 16oz. sirloin steak
- 4 tablespoons butter
- 1 ripe avocado
- Salt and pepper to taste

Directions:
1. Melt 2 tbsp. of butter in a huge skillet.
2. Fry eggs 4 at a time until the edges are crispy.
3. While the second batch of eggs are cooking, cook the sirloin in another skillet (with the other 2 tablespoons of butter) until it's at least 160°F.
4. Season eggs and steak well with salt and pepper.
5. Serve with slices of avocado.

Nutrition: Calories: 480 - Protein: 37g - Carbs: 4g - Fat: 37g – Fibre: 3g.

Chapter 8. Side Dishes

35.   Turkey and Cabbage Treat

Preparation Time: 5 minutes
Cooking time: 5 minutes
Servings: 4
Ingredients:

- 1 tablespoon lard, at room temperature
- 1/2 cup onion, chopped
- 1lb. ground turkey
- 10oz. puréed tomatoes
- Sea salt and ground black pepper, to taste
- 1 teaspoon cayenne pepper
- 1/4 teaspoon caraway seeds
- 1/4 teaspoon mustard seeds
- ½ lb. cabbage, cut into wedges
- 4 garlic cloves, minced
- 1 cup chicken broth
- 2 bay leaves

Directions:

1. Press the "Sauté" button to heat up your Instant Pot. Then, melt the lard. Cook the onion until translucent and tender.
2. Add ground turkey and cook until it is no longer pink; reserve the turkey/onion mixture.
3. Mix puréed tomatoes with salt, black pepper, cayenne pepper, caraway seeds, and mustard seeds.
4. Spritz the bottom and sides of the Instant Pot with a nonstick cooking spray. Then, place 1/2 of cabbage wedges on the bottom of your Instant Pot.
5. Spread the meat mixture over the top of the cabbage. Add minced garlic. Add the remaining cabbage.
6. Now, pour in the tomato mixture and chicken broth; lastly, add bay leaves.
7. Secure the lid. Choose "Manual" mode and High pressure; cook for 5 minutes. Once cooking is complete, use a natural pressure release; carefully remove the lid.

Nutrition: Calories: 247 - Fat: 12.5g - Carbs: 6.2g Protein: 25.3g - Sugars: 3.7g.

36.   Amazing Carrots Side Dish

Preparation time: 10 minutes
Cooking time: 10 minutes
Servings: 12
Ingredients:

- 3lb. carrots, peeled and cut into medium pieces
- A pinch of sea salt and black pepper
- ½ cup water
- ½ cup maple syrup
- 2 tablespoons olive oil
- ½ teaspoon orange rind, grated

Directions:

1. Put the oil in your instant pot, add the carrots and toss.
2. Add maple syrup, water, salt, pepper and orange rind, stir, cover and cook on High for 10 minutes.
3. Divide among plates and serve as a side dish.
4. Enjoy!

Nutrition: Calories: 140 - Fat: 2g - Fibre: 1g - Carbs: 2g - Protein: 6g.

37. Super Bowl with Eggplant and Chicken

Preparation Time: 3 minutes
Cooking Time: 8 minutes
Servings: 4
Ingredients:
- 1 tablespoon olive oil
- 1 leek, chopped
- 1lb.chicken breasts, diced
- 1lb. eggplant, peeled and sliced
- 1 teaspoon garlic paste
- 1/2 teaspoon turmeric powder
- 1 teaspoon red pepper flakes
- 1 cup broth, preferably homemade
- 1 cup tomatoes, puréed
- Kosher salt and ground black pepper, to taste

Directions:
1. Press the "Sauté" button to heat up your Instant Pot. Then, heat the oil. Cook the leeks until softened.
2. Now, add the chicken breasts; cook for 3 to 4 minute or until they are no longer pink. Then, add the remaining ingredients; stir to combine well.
3. Secure the lid. Choose "Poultry" mode and High pressure; cook for 5 minutes. Once cooking is complete, use a natural pressure release; carefully remove the lid.
4. Divide your dish among serving bowls and serve warm.

Nutrition: Calories: 317 - Fat: 20.9g - Carbs: 6.4g Protein: 22.9g - Sugars: 3.8g.

38. Great Side Dish

Preparation Time: 10 minutes
Cooking Time: 15 minutes
Servings: 3
Ingredients:
- 2 C. broccoli florets
- 1 small yellow onion, cut into wedges
- ½ tsp. garlic powder
- 1/8 tsp. paprika
- Freshly ground black pepper, to taste
- 1 tbsp. butter, melted

Directions:
1. Preheat the grill to medium heat.
2. In a large bowl, add all ingredients and toss to coat well.
3. Transfer the broccoli mixture over a double thickness of a foil paper.
4. Fold the foil around broccoli mixture to seal it.
5. Grill for about 10-15 minutes.
6. Serve hot.

Nutrition: Calories: 99 - Carbs: 6.5g - Protein: 2.1g - Fat: 7.9g - Sugar: 2.1g - Sodium: 76mg - Fibre: 2.1g.

39. Warm Chinese-Style Salad

Preparation Time: 2 minutes
Cooking Time: 8 minutes
Servings: 4
Ingredients:
- 2 tablespoons sesame oil
- 1 yellow onion, chopped
- 1 teaspoon garlic, finely minced
- 2-pound pe-tsai cabbage, shredded
- 1/4 cup rice wine vinegar
- 1/4 teaspoon Szechuan pepper
- 1/2 teaspoon salt
- 1 tablespoon soy sauce

Directions:
1. Press the "Sauté" button to heat up your Instant Pot. Then, heat the sesame oil. Cook the onion until softened.
2. Add the remaining ingredients.
3. Secure the lid. Choose "Manual" mode and High pressure; cook for 3 minutes. Once cooking is complete, use a quick pressure release; carefully remove the lid.
4. Transfer the cabbage mixture to a nice salad bowl and serve immediately.

Nutrition: Calories: 116 - Fat: 7.7g - Carbs: 6.2g Protein: 21g - Sugars: 3.3g.

40. Asparagus alla Fontina

Preparation Time: 2 minutes
Cooking Time: 8 minutes
Servings: 2
Ingredients:

- 1 tablespoon avocado oil
- 1/2lb. asparagus, trimmed
- 1/2 teaspoon celery salt
- 1/2 teaspoon cayenne pepper
- 1/4 teaspoon freshly ground black pepper
- 2 cloves garlic, crushed
- 2 (1-inch) piece ginger, grated
- 1 tablespoon coconut aminos
- 2 teaspoon dried basil
- 1/2 teaspoon dried oregano
- 1/2 cup Fontina cheese, grated
- 2 tablespoons fresh Italian parsley, roughly chopped

Directions:

1. Add all ingredients, except for cheese and parsley, to your Instant Pot.
2. Secure the lid. Choose "Manual" mode and High pressure; cook for 2 minutes. Once cooking is complete, use a quick pressure release; carefully remove the lid.
3. After that, top your asparagus with cheese and press the "Sauté" button. Allow it to simmer for 3 to 4 minutes or until cheese is melted.
4. Serve garnished with fresh parsley.

Nutrition: Calories: 223 - Fat: 17.5g - Carbs: 5.1g Protein: 11.4g - Sugars: 2.9g.

41. Quick and Easy Mushroom Casserole

Preparation Time: 5 minutes
Cooking Time: 10 minutes
Servings: 4
Ingredients:

- 2 tablespoons olive oil
- 2 chicken breasts, boneless, skinless and cut into slices
- Sea salt, to taste
- 1/4 teaspoon ground black pepper
- 1/2 teaspoon cayenne pepper
- 1 teaspoon fresh rosemary, finely minced
- 1 pound Portobello mushrooms, sliced
- 1/2 cup scallions, chopped
- 2 garlic cloves, minced
- 1 teaspoon yellow mustard
- 1 cup vegetable broth
- 1 tablespoon Piri-Piri sauce

Directions:

1. Press the "Sauté" button to heat up your Instant Pot. Then, heat the oil. Cook the chicken until delicately browned on all sides.
2. Season with salt, black pepper, cayenne pepper, and rosemary; reserve.
3. Spritz the bottom and sides of your Instant Pot with a nonstick cooking spray. Add 1/2 of the mushrooms to the bottom.
4. Add a layer of chopped scallions and minced garlic. Add the chicken mixture. Top with the remaining mushrooms.
5. In a mixing bowl, thoroughly combine vegetable broth and Piri-Piri sauce. Pour this sauce into the Instant Pot.
6. Secure the lid. Choose "Manual" mode and High pressure; cook for 5 minutes. Once cooking is complete, use a quick pressure release; carefully remove the lid. Serve warm and enjoy!

Nutrition: Calories: 229 - Fat: 10.6g - Carbs: 5.7g - Protein: 28g - Sugars: 2.6g.

42.   Easy Intermittent Steamed Salad

Preparation Time: 2 minutes
Cooking Time: 10 minutes
Servings: 4
Ingredients:
- 1 cup water
- 4 tomatoes, sliced
- 1 tablespoon extra-virgin olive oil
- 1/2 cup Halloumi cheese, crumbled
- 2 garlic cloves, smashed
- 2 tablespoons fresh basil, snipped

Directions:
1. Add 1 cup of water and a steamer rack to the Instant Pot.
2. Place the tomatoes on the steamer rack.
3. Secure the lid. Choose "Manual" mode and High pressure; cook for 3 minutes. Once cooking is complete, use a quick pressure release; carefully remove the lid.
4. Toss the tomatoes with the remaining ingredients and serve.

Nutrition: Calories: 168 - Fat: 12.4g - Carbs: 5.6g - Protein: 6.2g - Sugars: 3.5g.

43.   Zesty Brussels Sprout

Preparation Time: 15 minutes
Cooking Time: 15 minutes
Servings: 2
Ingredients:
- ½ lb. fresh Brussels sprouts, trimmed and halved
- 2 tbsp. olive oil
- 2 small garlic cloves, minced
- ½ tsp. red pepper flakes, crushed
- Salt and freshly ground black pepper, to taste
- 1 tbsp. fresh lemon juice
- 1 tsp. fresh lemon zest, grated finely

Directions:
1. Arrange a steamer basket over a large pan of the boiling water.
2. Place the asparagus into the steamer basket and steam, covered for about 6-8 minutes.

3. Remove from the heat and drain the asparagus well.
4. In a large skillet, heat the oil over medium heat and sauté the garlic and red pepper flakes for about 1 minute.
5. Stir in the Brussels sprouts, salt and black pepper and sauté for about 4-5 minutes.
6. Stir in the lemon juice and sauté for about 1 minute more.
7. Remove from the heat and serve hot with the garnishing of the lemon zest.

Nutrition: Calories: 116 - Carbs: 11g - Protein: 4.1g - Fat: 7.5g - Sugar: 2.5g; - Sodium: 102mg - Fibre: 4.4g.

44.   Buttered Broccoli

Preparation Time: 10 minutes
Cooking Time: 15 minutes
Servings: 4
Ingredients:
- 2 medium heads broccoli, cut into florets
- 2 garlic cloves, minced
- ¼ C. butter, melted
- 2 tbsp. fresh lemon juice
- 1 tsp. Italian seasoning
- Salt and freshly ground black pepper, to taste

Directions:
1. Preheat the oven to 450°F.
2. In a bowl, add all ingredients and toss to coat well.
3. Place broccoli mixture into a large baking dish and spread in a single layer.
4. Bake for about 12-15 minutes.
5. Serve hot.

Nutrition: Calories: 109 - Carbs: 7.4g - Protein: 3.1g - Fat: 12.3g - Sugar: 2g - Sodium: 155mg - Fibre: 2.6g.

45.   Appealing Broccoli Mash

Preparation Time: 15 minutes
Cooking Time: 5 minutes
Servings: 6
Ingredients:

- 16oz. broccoli florets
- 1 cup. water
- 1 tsp. fresh lemon juice
- 1 tsp. butter, softened
- 1 tsp. garlic, minced
- Salt and freshly ground black pepper, to taste

Directions:

1. In a medium pan, add the broccoli and water over medium heat and cook for about 5 minutes.
2. Drain the broccoli well and transfer into a large bowl
3. In the bowl of broccoli, add the lemon juice, butter, and garlic and with an immersion blender blend until smooth.
4. Season with salt and black pepper and serve.

Nutrition: Calories 32 - Carbs: 5.1g - Protein: 2g Fat: 0.9g - Sugar: 1.3g - Sodium: 160mg - Fibre: 2g.

46.   Simplest Yellow Squash

Preparation Time: 10 minutes
Cooking Time: 12 minutes
Servings: 4
Ingredients:

- 2 tbsp. olive oil
- 1 lb. yellow squash, cut into thin slices
- 1 small yellow onion, cut into thin rings
- 1 garlic clove, minced
- 3 tsp. water
- Salt and freshly ground white pepper, to taste

Directions:

1. In a large skillet, heat the oil over medium-high heat and stir fry the squash, onion and garlic for about 3-4 minutes.
2. Add water, salt and black pepper and stir to combine.

3. Reduce heat to low and simmer for about 6-8 minutes.
4. Serve hot.

Nutrition: Calories: 86 - Carbs: 5.7g - Protein: 1.6g - Fat: 7.2g - Sugar: 2.7g - Sodium: 51mg - Fibre: 1.7g.

47.   Pumpkin and Cauliflower Rice

Preparation time: 5 minutes
Cooking time: 10 minutes
Servings: 4
Ingredients:

- 2oz. olive oil
- 1 yellow onion, chopped
- 2 garlic cloves, minced
- 12oz. cauliflower rice
- 3 cups chicken stock
- 2oz. pumpkin puree
- ½ teaspoon nutmeg, ground
- 1 teaspoon thyme chopped
- ½ teaspoon ginger, grated
- ½ teaspoon cinnamon powder
- ½ teaspoon allspice
- 2oz. coconut cream

Directions:

1. Set your instant pot on sauté mode, add the oil, heat it up, add garlic and onion, stir and sauté for 3 minutes.
2. Add cauliflower rice, stock, pumpkin puree, thyme, nutmeg, cinnamon, ginger and allspice, stir, cover and cook on High for 12 minutes.
3. Add coconut cream, stir, divide among plates and serve as a side dish.

Nutrition: Calories: 15 - Fat: 2g - Fibre: 3g - Carbs: 5g - Protein: 6g.

48. Special Veggie Side Dish

Preparation time: 10 minutes
Cooking time: 12 minutes
Servings: 4
Ingredients:
- 2 cups cauliflower rice
- 1 cup mixed carrots and green beans
- 2 cups water
- ½ teaspoon green chilli, minced
- ½ teaspoon ginger, grated
- 3 garlic cloves, minced
- 2 tablespoons ghee
- 1 cinnamon stick
- 1 tablespoon cumin seeds
- 2 bay leaves
- 3 whole cloves
- Black peppercorns
- 2 whole cardamoms
- 1 tablespoon stevia
- A pinch of sea salt

Directions:
1. Put water in your instant pot, add cauliflower rice, mixed veggies, green chilli, grated ginger, garlic cloves, cinnamon stick, whole cloves and ghee and stir.
2. Also add cumin seeds, bay leaves, cardamoms, black peppercorns, salt and stevia, stir again, cover and cook on High for 12 minutes.
3. Discard cinnamon stick, bay leaves, cloves and cardamom, divide among plates and serve as a side dish.

Nutrition: Calories: 145 - Fat: 3g - Fibre: 1,5g - Carbs: 4g - Protein: 6g.

49. Great Broccoli Dish

Preparation time: 10 minutes
Cooking time: 12 minutes
Servings: 6
Ingredients:
- 31oz. broccoli florets
- 1 cup water
- Lemon slices
- A pinch of salt and black pepper

Directions:
1. Put the water in your instant pot, add the steamer basket, add broccoli florets and lemon slices, season with a pinch of salt and pepper, cover and cook on High for 12 minutes.
2. Divide among plates and serve as a side dish.

Nutrition: Calories: 152 - Fat: 2g - Fibre: 1g - Carbs: 2g - Protein: 3g.

50. Special Sweet Potatoes

Preparation time: 10 minutes
Cooking time: 10 minutes
Servings: 8
Ingredients:
- 1 cup water
- 1 tablespoon lemon peel, grated
- 2 tablespoons stevia
- A pinch of sea salt
- 2lb. sweet potatoes, peeled and sliced
- ¼ cup ghee
- ¼ cup maple syrup
- 1 cup pecans, chopped
- 1 tablespoon arrowroot powder
- Whole pecans for garnish

Directions:
1. Pour the water in your instant pot, add lemon peel, stevia, sweet potatoes and salt, stir, cover, cook on High for 10 minutes and transfer them to a plate.
2. Set your instant pot on Sauté mode, add the ghee and heat it up
3. Add pecans, maple syrup arrowroot powder, stir very well and cook for 1 minutes,
4. Divide sweet potatoes between plates, drizzle the pecans sauce all over, top with whole pecans and serve.

Nutrition: Calories: 162 - Fat: 2g - Fibre: 1g - Carbs: 5g - Protein 6g.

51. Brussels Sprouts Delight

Preparation time: 10 minutes
Cooking time: 8 minutes
Servings: 4
Ingredients:

- 2 tablespoons olive oil
- 2 garlic cloves, minced
- 2 tablespoons coconut aminos
- 1 and ½ pounds Brussels sprouts, halved
- 2oz. water
- 1 and ½ teaspoon white pepper

Directions:

1. Put the oil in your instant pot, add garlic, Brussels sprouts, aminos, water and white pepper, stir, cover and cook on High for 8 minutes.
2. Divide among plates and serve as a side dish.

Nutrition: Calories: 162 - Fat: 2g - Fibre: 1g - Carbs: 2g - Protein: 5g.

52. Tasty Cauliflower and Mint Rice

Preparation time: 10 minutes
Cooking time: 5 minutes
Servings: 4
Ingredients:

- 1 cup cauliflower rice
- 2 tablespoons olive oil
- 1 small yellow onion, chopped
- 1 and ½ cups veggie stock
- 2 tablespoons mint, chopped
- A pinch of salt and black pepper

Directions:

1. Set your instant pot on sauté mode, add the oil, heat it up, add onion, stir and cook for 3 minutes.
2. Add veggie stock, cauliflower rice, salt and pepper, stir, cover and cook on High for 5 minutes.
3. Add mint, toss everything to coat, divide between plates and serve right away as a side dish.

Nutrition: Calories: 160 - Fat: 3g - Fibre: 2g Carbs: 6g - Protein: 10g.

53. Instant Zucchini with Green Peppercorn Sauce

Preparation Time: 2 minutes
Cooking Time: 10 minutes
Servings: 4
Ingredients:

- 1 cup water
- 2 zucchinis, sliced
- Sea salt, to taste

Green Peppercorn Sauce:

- 2 tablespoons butter
- 1/2 cup green onions, minced
- 2 tablespoons Cognac
- 1 ½ cups chicken broth
- 1 cup whipping cream
- 1 ½ tablespoons green peppercorns in brine, drained and crushed slightly

Directions:

1. Add water and a steamer basket to the Instant Pot. Arrange your zucchini on the steamer basket.
2. Secure the lid. Choose "Manual" mode and Low pressure; cook for 3 minutes. Once cooking is complete, use a quick pressure release; carefully remove the lid.
3. Season zucchini with salt and set aside.
4. Wipe down the Instant Pot with a damp cloth. Press the "Sauté" button to heat up your Instant Pot.
5. Melt the butter and then, sauté green onions until tender. Add Cognac and cook for 2 minutes longer. Then, pour in chicken broth and let it boil another 4 minutes.
6. Lastly, stir in the cream and peppercorns. Continue to simmer until the sauce is thickened and thoroughly warmed.
7. Serve your zucchini with the sauce on the side.

Nutrition: Calories: 251 - Fat: 15.3g - Carbs: 3.2g Protein: 20.2g - Sugars: 1.5g.

54.   Stuffed Sausage with Bacon Wrappings

Preparation Time: 10 minutes
Cooking Time: 15 minutes
Servings: 4
Ingredients:

- Onion powder
- 8 bacon strips
- Salt.
- Garlic powder
- Black pepper
- 8 sausages
- ½ tsp Sweet paprika
- 16. pepper jack cheese slices

Directions:

1. Ensure you have a medium high source of heat. Set a grill on it. Add sausages to cook until done all sides and set on a plate to cool.
2. Slice a pocket opening in the sausages. Each to be stuffed with 2 slices of pepper jack cheese. Apply a seasoning of onion, pepper, garlic powder, paprika and salt.
3. Each stuffed sausage should be wrapped in a bacon strip and grip using a toothpick. Set them on the baking sheet and transfer to the oven to bake at 400°F for almost 15 minutes.
4. Serve immediately and enjoy.

Nutrition: Calories: 500 - Fat: 37g - Fibre: 12g - Carbs: 4g - Protein: 40g.

55.   Lazy Sunday Mushroom Ragout

Preparation Time: 2 minutes
Cooking Time: 10 minutes
Servings: 4
Ingredients:

- 2 tablespoons butter, at room temperature
- 1/2 cup white onions, peeled and sliced
- 1 cup chicken sausage, casing removed, sliced
- 1lb. chanterelle mushrooms, sliced
- 2 stalks spring garlic, diced
- Kosher salt and ground black pepper, to taste
- 1/2 teaspoon red pepper flakes
- 2 tablespoons tomato paste
- 1/2 cup good Pinot Noir
- 1 cup chicken stock
- 1/2 cup double cream
- 2 tablespoons fresh chives, chopped

Directions:

1. Press the "Sauté" button to heat up your Instant Pot. Once hot, melt the butter and sauté the onions until tender and translucent.
2. Add the sausage and mushrooms; continue to sauté until the sausage is no longer pink and the mushrooms are fragrant.
3. Then, stir in garlic and cook it for 30 to 40 seconds more or until aromatic. Now, add the salt, black pepper, red pepper, tomato paste, Pinot Noir, and chicken stock.
4. Secure the lid. Choose "Manual" mode and High pressure; cook for 5 minutes. Once cooking is complete, use a quick pressure release; carefully remove the lid.
5. After that, add double cream and press the "Sauté" button. Continue to simmer until everything is heated through and slightly thickened.
6. Lastly, divide your stew among individual bowls; top with fresh chopped chives and serve warm.

Nutrition: Calories: 279 - Fat: 2.3g - Carbs: 63g - Protein: 8.7g - Sugars: 3.2g.

56.   Special Collard Greens

Preparation time: 10 minutes
Cooking time: 5 minutes
Servings: 4
Ingredients:
- Olive oil
- 16oz. collard greens
- 1 cup yellow onion, chopped
- 2 garlic cloves, minced
- A pinch of sea salt and black pepper
- 14oz. veggie stock
- 1 bay leaf
- Tablespoon balsamic vinegar

Directions:
1. Set your instant pot on sauté mode, add the oil, heat it up, add onion, stir and sauté for 3 minutes.
2. Add collard greens, stir and sauté for 2 minutes more.
3. Add garlic, salt, pepper, stock and bay leaf, stir, cover and cook on High for 5 minutes.
4. Add vinegar, toss, divide among plates and serve.

Nutrition: Calories: 130 - Fat: 1g - Fibre: 2g Carbs: 3g - Protein 5g.

57.   Rolls of Sausage Pizzas

Preparation Time: 10 minutes
Cooking Time: 30 minutes
Servings: 6
Ingredients:
- ¼ cup. pizza sauce,
- 2 cups. shredded mozzarella cheese,
- ½ cup. cooked sausage,
- Salt.
- 1 tsp. pizza seasoning,
- 2 tbsps. chopped onion,
- Black pepper.
- ¼ cup. chopped red and green bell peppers,
- 1 chopped tomato,

Directions:
1. Line a baking sheet. Grease it slightly. Over the sheet, spread mozzarella cheese and top with sprinkles of pizza seasoning. Set in an oven preheated to 400°F and bake until done for 20 minutes.
2. Remove the pizza crust from the oven. Spread it with tomatoes, sausage, bell peppers and onion. Top with tomato sauce drizzling.
3. Put it back at the oven and bake for another 10 minutes.
4. Remove the pizza from oven and allow to cool. Slice into 6 equal parts and roll. Enjoy your lunch.

Nutrition: Calories: 117 - Fibre: 1g - Carbs: 2g - Fat: 7g - Protein: 11g.

58.   Coated Avocado Tacos

Preparation Time: 10 minutes
Cooking Time: 20 minutes
Servings: 12
Ingredients:
- 1 avocado
- Tortillas and toppings
- ½ cup panko breadcrumbs
- 1 egg
- Salt

Directions:
1. Scoop out the meat from each avocado shell and slice them into wedges.
2. Beat the egg in a shallow bowl and put the breadcrumbs in another bowl.
3. Dip the avocado wedges in the beaten egg and coat with breadcrumbs. Sprinkle them with a bit of salt. Arrange them in the cooking basket in a single layer.
4. Cook for 15 minutes at 400°F. Shake the basket halfway in the cooking process.
5. Put the cooked avocado wedges in tortillas and add your preferred toppings.

Nutrition: Calories: 179 - Fat: 6.1g - Carbs: 26.3g - Protein: 4.9g.

59.　　Potato Bites

Preparation Time: 2 minutes
Cooking Time: 12 minutes
Servings: 4
Ingredients:
- 2 tsp. olive oil
- 2 lb. sliced potatoes
- Black pepper
- ¼ tsp. salt

Directions:
1. Preheat Pan to a temperature of 370°F.
2. Sprinkle salt and pepper on potatoes and drizzle olive oil.
3. Transfer into Pan basket and cook for 12 minutes.
4. Shake the basket of fryer after every 2 minutes then serve.

Nutrition: Calories: 184 - Protein: 4.3g - Fat: 2.44g - Carbs: 37.21g.

60.　　Roasted Sweet Carrots

Preparation Time: 2 minutes
Cooking Time: 8 minutes
Servings: 4
Ingredients:
- 1lb. sliced carrots
- ¼ tsp. white pepper
- 2 tbsps. lime juice
- 2 tbsps. of honey
- ¼ tsp of salt

Directions:
1. Preheat Pan to a temperature of 350°F.
2. In a bowl add honey, salt, pepper, and lime juice, mix.
3. Now add carrots and toss to combine.
4. Place carrots into fryer basket and cook for 8 minutes.
5. Serve!

Nutrition: Calories: 113 - Protein: 1.2g - Fat: 0.28g - Carbs: 28.9g.

61.　　Crispy Potato Skins

Preparation Time: 5 minutes
Cooking Time: 55 minutes
Servings: 2
Ingredients:
- 2 Yukon Gold potatoes
- ¼ tsp. sea salt
- ½ tsp. olive oil
- 2 minced green onions
- 4 bacon strips
- ¼ cup shredded cheddar cheese
- 1/3 cup sour cream

Directions:
1. Rinse and scrub the potatoes until clean. Rub with oil and sprinkle with salt. Put them in the cooking basket. Cook for 35 minutes at 400°F. Transfer the cooked potatoes to a platter.
2. Put the bacon strip in the cooking basket. Cook for 5 minutes at 400°F.
3. Move to a plate and leave to cool. Crumble into bits.
4. Slice the potatoes in half.
5. Scoop out most of the meat.
6. Arrange the potato skins with the skin facing side up in the cooking basket. Spray them with oil.
7. Cook for 3 minutes at 400°F. Flip the potato skins.
8. Fill each piece with cheese and crumbled bacon. Continue cooking for 2 more minutes.
9. Transfer to a platter. Add a little portion of sour cream on top. Sprinkle with minced onion and serve while warm.

Nutrition: Calories: 483 - Fat: 8.7g - Carbs: 92.8g - Protein: 12.5g.

62. Roasted Corn with Butter and Lime

Preparation Time: 2 minutes
Cooking Time: 20 minutes
Servings: 4
Ingredients:
- 4 ears corn
- ½ tsp. pepper
- 1 tsp. lime juice
- 1 tbsp. chopped parsley
- 1 tbsp. butter
- ¼ tsp. salt

Directions:
1. Preheat Pan to a temperature of 400°F
2. Remove husk and transfer corns into Pan and cook for 20 minutes.
3. After every 5 minutes shake the fryer basket.
4. When done rub butter.
5. Sprinkle parsley, pepper, and salt.
6. Drizzle lime juice on top, serve.

Nutrition: Calories: 114 - Protein: 3.4g - Fat: 4.26g - Carbs: 19.24g.

63. Coconut Gratin

Preparation Time: 10 minutes
Cooking Time: 50 minutes
Servings: 8
Ingredients:
- 2 tablespoons olive oil
- 2 garlic cloves, minced
- 1 tablespoon balsamic vinegar
- 1/3 cup coconut cream
- A pinch of salt and black pepper
- 2 tablespoons marjoram, chopped
- ½ cup parmesan, grated
- 3lb. tomatoes, sliced
- Cooking spray

Directions:
1. Heat up a pan with the olive oil over medium heat, add the garlic, stir and cook for 2 minutes.
2. Add the vinegar, coconut cream, salt, pepper and marjoram, stir and cook for 3 minutes more.
3. Grease baking dish with cooking spray and arrange the tomato slices.

4. Pour the coconut cream mix all over, spread, sprinkle parmesan on top, introduce in the oven and bake at 400°F for 45 minutes.
5. Divide the gratin between plates and serve as a side dish.

Nutrition: Calories: 251- Fat: 3g - Fibre: 7g - Carbs: 12g - Protein: 9g.

64. Maple Syrup Bacon

Preparation Time: 5 minutes
Cooking Time: 10 minutes
Servings: 2
Ingredients:
- Maple syrup.
- 11 thick bacon slices.

Directions:
1. Preheat your pan to 400°F.
2. Place the bacon on the flat surface and brush with the maple syrup.
3. Move to the pan to cook for 10 minutes.
4. Serve and enjoy!

Nutrition: Calories: 91 - Carbs: 0g - Protein: 8g - Fat: 2g.

65. Celery and Chilli Peppers Stir Fry

Preparation Time: 10 minutes
Cooking Time: 5 minutes
Servings: 6
Ingredients:
- 2 tablespoons olive oil
- Chilli peppers, dried and crushed
- 2 cups celery, julienned
- 2 tablespoons coconut aminos

Directions:
1. Heat up a pan with the oil at medium-high heat, add chilli peppers, stir and cook them for 2 minutes.
2. Add the celery and the coconut aminos, stir, cook for 3 minutes more, divide between plates and serve as a side dish.

Nutrition: Calories:162 - Fat: 2g - Fibre: 7g - Carbs: 12g - Protein: 7g

Chapter 9. First Courses

66.   Celery and Mozzarella Side Salad

Preparation Time: 10 minutes
Cooking Time: 0 minutes
Servings: 4
Ingredients:
- 7oz. mozzarella, shredded
- 2 cups cherry tomatoes, halved
- 2 celery stalks, chopped
- Juice of 1 lemon
- 2 tablespoons olive oil
- A pinch of salt and black pepper
- ½ teaspoon oregano, dried

Directions:
1. In a bowl, place and combine the tomatoes with the celery, oregano, mozzarella, lemon juice, salt, pepper and the oil, toss, divide between plates then serve.

Nutrition: Calories: 100 - Fat: 2g - Fibre: 4g - Carbs: 9g - Protein: 6g.

67.   Mustard Cabbage

Preparation Time: 10 minutes
Cooking Time: 20 minutes
Servings: 4
Ingredients:
- 1 onion, sliced
- 1 cabbage head, shredded
- A pinch of salt and black pepper
- 1 cup chicken stock
- 2 tablespoons mustard
- 1 tablespoon olive oil

Directions:
1. Heat up a pan with the oil at medium-high heat, add the onion, stir and cook for 5 minutes.
2. Add the cabbage, salt, pepper, stock and mustard, stir, cook for 15 minutes, divide between plates and serve as a side dish.

Nutrition: Calories: 197 - Fat: 4g - Fibre: 2g - Carbs: 8g - Protein: 5g.

68.   Lemon Parsnips Mix

Preparation Time: 10 minutes
Cooking Time: 35 minutes
Servings: 6
Ingredients:
- 1lb. parsnips, cut into medium chunks
- 2 tablespoons lemon peel, grated
- 1 cup veggie stock
- A pinch of salt and black pepper
- Olive oil
- ¼ cup cilantro, chopped

Directions:
1. Heat up a pan with the oil at medium-high heat, add the parsnips, stir and brown them for 5 minutes.
2. Add lemon peel, stock, salt, pepper and cilantro, stir, cover the pan, reduce heat to medium and cook for 30 minutes.
3. Divide the mix between then serve.

Nutrition: Calories: 179 - Fat: 4g - Fibre: 4g - Carbs: 6g - Protein: 8g.

69.   Squash Wedges

Preparation Time: 10 minutes
Cooking Time: 10 minutes
Servings: 4
Ingredients:
- 1lb. butternut squash, cut into medium wedges
- Olive oil for frying
- A pinch of salt and black pepper
- ¼ teaspoon baking soda

Directions:
1. Heat a pan with olive oil at medium-high heat, put squash wedges, season with salt, pepper and the baking soda, cook until they are gold on all sides, drain grease, divide between plates then serve.

Nutrition: Calories: 202 - Fat: 5g - Fibre: 5g - Carbs: 7g - Protein: 11g.

70. Radish and Cabbage Mix

Preparation Time: 40 minutes
Cooking Time: 15 minutes
Servings: 6
Ingredients:
- Salt and black pepper to the taste
- 1 pound napa cabbage, chopped
- 2 cups veggie stock
- 1 cup radish, chopped
- 1 garlic clove, minced
- 1 green onion stalks, chopped
- 1 tablespoon coconut aminos
- 2 tablespoons chilli flakes
- 1 tablespoon olive oil

Directions:
1. In a bowl, mix the cabbage with salt and black pepper, massage well for 10 minutes, cover and leave aside for 30 minutes.
2. In another bowl, mix chilli flakes with aminos, garlic and oil and whisk well.
3. Heat up a pan with the chilli mix over medium-high heat, add the cabbage, stock and radish, stir, cover and cook for 15 minutes.
4. Divide between plates then serve.

Nutrition: Calories: 200 - Fat:3g - Fibre: 4g - Carbs: 15g - Protein: 8g.

71. Walnuts Broccoli Salad

Preparation Time: 10 minutes
Cooking Time: 20 minutes
Servings: 6
Ingredients:
- 3 cups broccoli florets
- 14oz. tomato paste
- 1 tablespoon olive oil
- 1 yellow onion, chopped
- 1 teaspoon thyme, dried
- Salt and black pepper to the taste
- ½ cup walnuts, chopped

Directions:
1. Heat up a pan with the oil at medium-high heat, add the onion, stir and cook for 5 minutes.
2. Add broccoli, tomato paste, thyme, salt and pepper, toss, cook for 10 minutes, divide between plates, sprinkle walnuts on top and serve as a side dish.

Nutrition: Calories: 197 - Fat: 12g - Fibre: 2g - Carbs: 7g - Protein: 7g.

72. Cabbage Sauté

Preparation Time: 5 minutes
Cooking Time: 10 minutes
Servings: 2
Ingredients:
- 6oz. kale
- 6oz. green cabbage
- 6oz. red cabbage
- 1 tablespoon lemon juice
- 2 tablespoons olive oil
- ¼ teaspoon black pepper
- Salt to taste

Directions:
1. Tear the kale leaves from stems and cut the cabbage into thin pieces.
2. Take a skillet and heat the oil over a low to medium heat. Put everything into a skillet. Pour some lemon juice and season the mixture with some salt and pepper. Stir everything together.
3. Leave the skillet over medium heat and cook the mixture for 5-10 minutes or until you notice it became tender and golden at the edges.

Nutrition: Calories: 148 - Carbs: 4g - Fibre: 2g - Fat: 14g - Protein: 1.7g.

73.   Paprika Green Cabbage

Preparation Time: 10 minutes
Cooking Time: 20 minutes
Servings: 4
Ingredients:

- 1 and ½ pound green cabbage, shredded
- Salt and black pepper to the taste
- 2 tablespoons olive oil
- 1 tablespoon parsley, chopped
- 1 cup veggie stock
- ¼ teaspoon sweet paprika

Directions:

1. Heat up a pan with the oil at medium-high heat, add cabbage, salt, pepper, paprika and stock, stir and cook for 20 minutes.
2. Add the parsley, stir, divide between plates and serve as a side dish.

Nutrition: Calories: 200 - Fat: 4g - Fibre: 2g - Carbs:14g - Protein: 5g.

74.   Celery Mix

Preparation Time: 10 minutes
Cooking Time: 20 minutes
Servings: 4
Ingredients:

- 1lb. celery, peeled and cubed
- 1 garlic clove, minced
- Salt and black pepper to the taste
- 1 tablespoon rosemary, chopped
- 1 tablespoon avocado oil

Directions:

1. Heat up a pan with the oil at medium-high heat, add the celery, stir and cook for 5 minutes.
2. Add garlic, salt, pepper and rosemary, stir, cook for 15 minutes more, divide between plates and serve as a side dish.

Nutrition: Calories: 200 - Fat: 3g - Fibre: 3g - Carbs: 8g - Protein: 9g.

75.   Acorn Squash Puree

Preparation Time: 5 minutes
Cooking Time: 45 minutes
Servings: 6
Ingredients:

- 1 acorn squash
- 1 tablespoon extra-virgin olive oil

Directions:

1. Preheat the oven to 350°F.
2. Start by cutting the vegetable lengthwise on a cutting board. Take a spoon and dig out all the seeds and strings. Discard or save the seeds for roasting later on.
3. Take a basting brush and dip it in extra-virgin olive oil. Evenly spread the oil over the entire vegetable.
4. Place the vegetable flesh down on a cookie sheet lined with aluminum foil. You want the hard shell to be face up when roasting.
5. Bake in the oven for 45 minutes. When done, remove the cookie sheet from the oven and let it cool for about 10 minutes.
6. Flip it over and grab a spoon. Dig out the cooked squash and place into a food processor. Note: It should be extremely tender and easy to spoon out.
7. Turn on the food processor or blender and puree for 20-30 seconds.
8. Serve immediately.

Nutrition: Calories: 49 - Fat: 2g - Fibre: 1g - Carbs: 7g - Protein: 1g.

76. Creamy Cabbage

Preparation Time: 5 minutes
Cooking Time: 10 minutes
Servings: 2
Ingredients:

- 1lb. cabbage
- 1 garlic clove
- 1 tablespoon butter (or coconut oil)
- 1oz. vegetable broth (or water)
- 1 ½ ounces heavy cream (or coconut cream)
- Salt to taste

Directions:

1. Cut the cabbage into thin slices and crush the garlic.
2. Take a large skillet and melt the butter over medium-high heat. Add in cabbage and garlic and cook for 3-4 minutes until you notice cabbage got tender.
3. Pour the broth and cream to the skillet and stir everything together. Wait until everything simmers and then cook it for 3-4 more minutes. You will know you are done when the cream is thick, and the cabbage is softer. Serve the meal while it's hot.

Nutrition: Calories: 149 - Fibre: 1.6g - Carbs: 4.4g - Fat: 14.3g - Protein: 1.9g.

77. Creamy Coleslaw

Preparation Time: 10 minutes
Cooking Time: 2 minutes
Servings: 2
Ingredients:

- 4oz. green cabbage
- 1oz. red cabbage
- 1 cucumber
- Black olives
- 1 tablespoon scallions
- 2 tablespoons mayonnaise
- ½ tablespoon lemon juice
- 1 tablespoon dill
- 1 tablespoon parsley
- Salt to taste

Directions:

1. Cut the red and green cabbage, olives, scallions, and cucumber into bite-sized pieces and add them to a bowl. Add some salt.
2. Put the lemon juice and mayo in another bowl. Mince the parsley and dill and combine them in.
3. Mix the wet and dry ingredients so you can prepare coleslaw. You can wait for the mixture to marinate a little bit and leave it aside for an hour or simply serve it right away

Nutrition: Calories: 222 - Carbs: 4g - Fibre: 2g - Fat: 21g - Protein: 1.5g.

78. Crispy Bacon and Kale

Preparation Time: 5 minutes
Cooking Time: 14 minutes
Servings: 2
Ingredients:

- 1 ½ ounces bacon
- 4oz. kale
- ¼ teaspoon black pepper
- Salt to taste

Directions:

1. Take a wide pot (that will be suitable for kale you'll add later) and add bacon. Cook the strips over medium heat until they become crispy. Put them aside.
2. Lower the heat, cut your kale and place it in the pot. Cook the kale on the bacon grease for 5 minutes or until it becomes wilted. Toss in some pepper and salt.
3. Slice the bacon into smaller pieces and mix it with the kale. Serve it warm!

Nutrition: Calories: 116 - Carbs: 2.5g - Fibre: 1.2g - Fat: 7.7g - Protein: 8.3g.

79. Coconut, Green Beans & Shrimp Curry Soup

Preparation Time: 10 minutes
Cooking Time: 15 minutes
Servings: 4
Ingredients:
- 1tbsp. ghee
- 1 lb. jumbo shrimp, peeled and deveined
- 1tsp ginger-garlic puree
- 1tbsp. red curry paste
- 1 ½ cup coconut milk
- Salt and chilli pepper to taste
- 1 bunch green beans, halved

Directions:
1. Melt ghee in a medium saucepan over medium heat. Add the shrimp, season with salt and black pepper, and cook until they are opaque, 2 to 3 minutes. Remove shrimp to a plate. Add the ginger-garlic puree and red curry paste to the ghee and sauté for 2 minutes until fragrant.
2. Stir in the coconut milk; add the shrimp, salt, chilli pepper, and green beans. Cook for 4 minutes. Reduce the heat to a simmer and cook an additional 3 minutes, occasionally stirring. Adjust taste with salt, fetch soup into serving bowls, and serve with cauli rice.

Nutrition: Calories: 375 - Fat: 35.4g - Carbs: 2g - Protein: 9g.

80. Salsa Verde Chicken Soup

Preparation Time: 5 minutes
Cooking Time: 10 minutes
Servings: 4
Ingredients:
- ½ cup salsa Verde
- 2 cups cooked and shredded chicken
- 2 cups chicken broth
- 1 cup shredded cheddar cheese
- 3oz. cream cheese
- ½ tsp chilli powder
- ½ tsp ground cumin
- ½ tsp fresh cilantro, chopped
- Salt and black pepper, to taste

Directions:
1. Combine the cream cheese, salsa Verde, and broth, in a food processor; pulse until smooth. Transfer the mixture to a pot and place over medium heat.
2. Cook until hot, but do not bring to a boil. Add chicken, chilli powder, and cumin and cook for about 3-5 minutes, or until it is heated through.
3. Stir in cheddar cheese and season with salt and pepper to taste. If it is very thick, add a few tablespoons of water and boil for 1-3 more minutes. Serve hot in bowls sprinkled with fresh cilantro.

Nutrition: Calories: 346 - Fat: 23g - Carbs: 3g - Protein: 25g.

81. Creamy Squash Soup

Preparation Time: 15 minutes
Cooking Time: 30 minutes
Servings: 4
Ingredients:
- 2lb. butternut squash, cubed
- 1 tbsp. olive oil
- 1 onion, chopped
- Cloves garlic, minced
- 1 ½ tsp. salt
- ½ tsp. black pepper
- 25.7oz. vegetable stock
- 3.5oz. heavy cream

Directions:
1. Heat the oil in a heavy skillet over medium-high heat. Add onion, garlic, salt, pepper, and sauté, stirring, until the onion is translucent.
2. Add squash and stock to a large pot. Transfer vegetables to the pot.
3. Bring to a low simmer and cook until the squash is tender, about 20-30 minutes. Add water if necessary, during cooking.
4. Add the cream, stirring to combine. If you have an immersion blender, use it to puree the soup in the pot. If not, transfer the soup to a blender or food processor and blend to a smooth puree.
5. Serve warm.

Nutrition: Calories: 205- Fat: 22g - Carbs: 9g - Protein: 3g.

82. Sicilian-Style Zoodle Spaghetti

Preparation time: 5 minutes
Cooking time: 15 minutes
Servings: 4
Ingredients:
- 1 cup zoodles (spiraled zucchini)
- 8oz. cubed bacon
- 3.5oz. canned sardines, chopped
- ½ cup canned chopped tomatoes
- 1 tbsp capers
- 1 tbsp parsley
- 1 tsp minced garlic

Directions:
1. Pour some of the sardine oil in a pan. Add garlic and cook for 1 minute. Add the bacon and cook for 2 more minutes. Stir in the tomatoes and let simmer for 5 minutes. Add zoodles and sardines and cook for 3 minutes.

Nutrition: Calories: 355 - Fat: 31g - Carbs: 6g - Protein: 20g.

83. Intermittent Vegetarian Chilli

Preparation Time: 15 minutes
Cooking Time: 35 minutes
Servings: 2
Ingredients:
- ½ lbs. ground beef, 85 percent lean
- ½ large white onion, diced
- 1 cloves garlic, minced
- 1 can (15 oz.) diced tomatoes, liquid reserved
- 1oz. tomato paste
- 1oz. canned green chillies, liquid reserved
- 1 tbsp. Worcestershire sauce
- Chilli powder
- 1 tbsp. cumin
- 1 Tbsp. dried oregano
- 1 tsp. kosher salt
- 1 tsp. freshly ground black pepper
- 1 tbsp. olive oil

Directions:
1. Heat the oil in a heavy stockpot over medium-high heat. When the oil is hot, add the onions and sauté until soft and translucent, about 5 minutes.
2. Add garlic to the pot and sauté for one minute more.
3. Add the rest of the ingredients to the pot and stir to combine.
4. Bring to a low simmer and cook until fragrant, about 30 minutes. Add water if necessary, during cooking.

Nutrition: Calories: 476 - Fat: 18g - Carbs: 13g - Protein: 23g.

84. Creamy Intermittent Broccoli Cheese Soup

Preparation Time: 5 minutes
Cooking Time: 35 minutes
Servings: 2
Ingredients:
- 1 cup broccoli, chopped
- 2oz. cheddar cheese, grated
- 1 tbsp. butter
- ¼ cup onion, diced
- ¼ cup celery, diced
- 1 ½ cups vegetable stock
- ½ cup heavy cream
- 1 tbsp. olive oil

Directions:
1. Heat the oil in a heavy stockpot over medium-high heat. When the oil is hot, add the onions and celery to the pot and sauté until the onion is soft and translucent, about 5 minutes.
2. Add garlic to the pot and sauté for one minute more.
3. Add the rest of the ingredients, excluding the cream and cheese, to the pot and stir to combine.
4. Bring to a low simmer and cook until the vegetables are tender, about 30 minutes. Add water if necessary during cooking.
5. Stir in cream, stirring constantly until the cheese is melted and soup is thick and creamy.
6. Transfer to serving bowls and serve hot.

Nutrition: Calories: 333 - Fat: 36g - Carbs: 5g - Protein: 13g.

85.	Intermittent Mexican-Style Soup

Preparation Time: 10 minutes
Cooking Time: 40 minutes
Servings: 8-10
Ingredients:

- ¼ cup onion, diced
- Cloves garlic, minced
- 1Tbsp. chilli powder
- 1 tsp. cumin
- 20oz. canned diced tomatoes
- 2oz. canned green chillies
- 32oz.ground beef
- 3oz. cream cheese
- ½ cup heavy cream
- 1 tbsp. olive oil

Directions:

1. Heat the oil in a heavy stockpot over medium-high heat. When the oil is hot, add the onions to the pot and sauté until soft and translucent, about 5 minutes.
2. Add garlic to the pot and sauté for one minute more.
3. Add ground beef to the pot and sauté until the meat is thoroughly browned, stirring constantly with a wooden spoon or spatula. This should take about 10 minutes.
4. Add the rest of the ingredients, excluding the cream and cream cheese, to the pot and stir to combine.
5. Bring to a low simmer and cook until fragrant, about 30 minutes. Add water if necessary during cooking.
6. Stir in cream and cream cheese, stirring constantly until cream cheese is melted and soup is thick and creamy.
7. Transfer to serving bowls and serve hot.

Nutrition: Calories: 450 - Fat: 28g - Carbs: 8g - Protein: 27g.

86.	Zoodles With White Clam Sauce

Preparation time: 10 minutes
Cooking time: 19 minutes
Servings: 2
Ingredients:

- 1 tsp kosher salt
- ¼ cup butter
- 1 tbsp minced garlic
- 2 tbsp olive oil
- ¼ tsp ground black pepper
- ½ cup dry white wine
- Drained baby clams (1 large can)
- Chopped parsley
- 2 tbsp lemon juice
- 1 lb. zucchini noodles
- 1 tsp grated lemon zest

Directions:

1. Mix the olive oil, pepper, butter and salt in a large pan that is set over medium heat. When they're all mixed up, add your minced garlic and let that cook for 2 minutes.
2. Now add your white wine and lemon juice and let that cook for two minutes or until the size of the mix slightly reduced.
3. Done? Good. Now throw in your clams and let them cook until they open up. Throw away any that refuse to open, say no to stubborn clams!
4. When all the clams are open, remove from heat and add your noodles. Coat the noodles in the clam sauce and leave it to soften for about 2 minutes.
5. Add parsley and grated lemon zest and stir. Taste for seasoning and add more salt if you like.

Nutrition: Calories: 311 - Fat: 19g - Carbs: 9g - Protein :13g - Fibre :2g.

87. Intermittent Yellow Curry

Preparation Time: 10 minutes
Cooking Time: 30 minutes
Servings: 2
Ingredients:

- 14oz. can unsweetened coconut milk, full fat
- 1tsp. Thai yellow curry paste
- 1tsp. soy sauce
- 1 tsp. honey
- 1 green onion chopped
- 1 cloves garlic, minced
- 1 tbsp. fresh ginger, minced
- ¼ cup fresh cilantro, chopped
- ¼ cup spring onions, chopped

Directions:

1. Place coconut milk, curry paste, soy sauce and honey into a heavy stock pot.
2. Bring to a low simmer and cook until the spices are fragrant, about 30 minutes. Add water if necessary during cooking.
3. Transfer to serving bowls and garnish with cilantro and spring onions.
4. Serve hot.

Nutrition Calories: 25 - Fat: 29g - Carbs: 9g - Protein: 14g.

88. Sour Cream Salmon with Parmesan

Preparation time: 5 minutes
Cooking time: 25 minutes
Servings: 4
Ingredients:

- 1 cup sour cream
- ½ tbsp minced dill
- ½ lemon, zested and juiced
- Pink salt and black pepper to season
- (4 pieces)21oz. salmon steaks
- ½ cup grated Parmesan cheese

Directions:

1. Preheat oven to 400°F and line a baking sheet with parchment paper; set aside. In a bowl, mix the sour cream, dill, lemon zest, juice, salt and black pepper, and set aside.
2. Season the fish with salt and black pepper, drizzle lemon juice on both sides

of the fish and arrange them in the baking sheet. Spread the sour cream mixture on each fish and sprinkle with Parmesan.

3. Bake the fish for 15 minutes and after broil the top for 2 minutes with a close watch for a nice a brown color. Plate the fish and serve with buttery green beans.

Nutrition: Calories: 288 - Fat 23.4g - Carbs 1.2g Protein 16.2g.

89. Intermittent Chinese-Style Soup

Preparation Time: 5 minutes
Cooking Time: 35 minutes
Servings: 6
Ingredients:

- 2 cups vegetable stock
- 1lb. pork tenderloin or other lean pork, sliced into thin bite-sized pieces
- 1 cup fresh mushrooms, chopped
- 1tbsp. soy sauce
- 1 tbsp. white vinegar
- 1tbsp. rice vinegar
- 1 tsp. salt
- 1tsp. freshly ground black pepper
- 1tbsp. water
- 3 eggs, beaten
- 1lb. tofu, extra firm, cubed

Directions:

1. Put all ingredients, excluding eggs and tofu, in a heavy stock pot.
2. Bring to a low simmer and cook until the meat is thoroughly cooked and the mushrooms are tender, about 30 minutes. Add water if necessary during cooking.
3. Slowly and carefully, stir in the tofu and beaten eggs. Allow the warm soup to sit for at least 3 minute to allow the eggs to cook.
4. Transfer to serving bowls and serve hot.

Nutrition: Calories: 150 - Fat: 5g - Carbs: 5g - Protein: 20g.

Chapter 10. Meat

90.   Seasoned Pork Chops

Preparation time: 10 minutes
Cooking time: 15 minutes
Servings: 8
Ingredients:
- 2 garlic cloves, minced
- Freshly ground black pepper, to taste
- 1 lime, juiced
- 1 tablespoon fresh basil, chopped
- 1 tablespoon Old Bay seafood seasoning
- ½ cup apple cider vinegar
- ½ cup olive oil
- 8 boneless pork chops, cut into ½ inch thick

Directions:
1. Add the minced garlic, black pepper, lime juice, basil, seasoning, apple cider vinegar, and olive oil to a Ziploc bag.
2. Place the pork chops in this bag and seal it. Shake it well to coat the pork and place it in the refrigerator for 6 hours. Continue flipping and shaking the bag every 1 hour.
3. Meanwhile, preheat your outdoor grill over medium-high heat.
4. Remove the pork chops from the Ziploc bag and discard its marinade.
5. Grill all the marinated pork chops for 7 minutes per side until their internal temperature reaches 145°F. Serve warm on a plate.

Nutrition: Calories: 412 - Fat: 26.4g - Carbs: 1.0g - Fibre: 0.1g - Protein: 40g.

91.   Garlicky Pork Roast

Preparation time: 20 minutes
Cooking time: 2 hours
Servings: 6
Ingredients:
- 2 ½ lb. pork tenderloin
- 2 garlic cloves, minced
- 1 tablespoon olive oil

- 2 tablespoons dried rosemary

Directions:
1. Preheat the oven to 375°F.
2. Mix the garlic, olive oil, and rosemary in a bowl, then rub this mixture all over the pork tenderloin.
3. Place the pork tenderloin in a roasting pan and roast in the preheated oven for about 2 hours, or until the internal temperature reaches 145°F.
4. Once roasted, remove the tenderloin from the oven. Slice and serve warm.

Nutrition: Calories: 274 - Fat: 7.4g - Total Carbs: 1.4g - Fibre: 0.7g - Protein: 47.7g.

92.   Spiced Pork Tenderloin

Preparation time: 10 minutes
Cooking time: 2 hours
Servings: 4
Ingredients:
- 2 teaspoons minced garlic
- 1 tablespoon fresh cilantro
- 1 dash ground black pepper
- 2½ teaspoons ground cumin
- 1 teaspoon salt
- 1 tablespoon chilli powder
- 2lb. pork tenderloin, cubed

Directions:
1. In a bowl, add the garlic, cilantro, black pepper, cumin, salt, and chilli powder. Mix these spices together.
2. Toss in the pork cubes and coat them well with the spice mixture.
3. Cover the pork cubes and refrigerate them for 45 minutes to marinate.
4. Meanwhile, preheat the oven to 225°F.
5. Arrange the spiced pork in a baking tray and roast for 2 hours, or until crispy.
6. Remove from the oven and serve on a plate.

Nutrition: Calories: 291 - Fat: 8.9g - Total Carbs: 3.1g - Fibre: 1.6g - Protein: 47.7g.

93. Kalamata Parsley Tapenade and Salted Lamp Chops

Preparation time: 15 minutes
Cooking time: 25 minutes
Servings: 4
Ingredients:
Tapenade:

- 1 cup pitted Kalamata olive
- 2 teaspoons minced garlic
- 2 tablespoons extra-virgin olive oil
- 1 tablespoon chopped fresh parsley
- 2 teaspoons freshly squeezed lemon juice

Lamb chops:

- 1lb. racks French-cut lamb chops (8 bones each)
- Sea salt and ground black pepper, to taste
- 1 tablespoon olive oil

Directions:

1. Make the tapenade:
2. In a food processor, add the olives, garlic, olive oil, parsley, and lemon juice and blend well until it becomes slightly chunky purée.
3. Add the purée in a container. Cover with a plastic wrap and reserve in the refrigerator until ready to use.
4. Make the lamb chops:
5. Preheat the oven to 450°F.
6. Sprinkle the lamb racks with salt and pepper.
7. Heat olive oil in a skillet over medium-high heat. Sear for about 5 minutes until the lamb racks are browned. Flip the lamb racks halfway through the cooking time.
8. Turn the racks and interlace the bones. Roast in the preheated oven for about 20 minutes to get medium-rare results.
9. Allow the lamb to rest for about 10 minutes, then slice into chops.
10. Serve the chops equally to 4 plates, then top with the tapenade before serving.

Nutrition: Calories: 347 - Fat: 27g - Total Carbs: 2.0g - Fibre: 1.0g - Protein: 20g.

94. Sausage, Beef and Chilli Recipe

Preparation time: 20 minutes
Cooking time: 8 hours
Servings: 6
Ingredients:

- 1lb. mild bulk sausage
- 1lb. ground beef
- 2 minced cloves garlic
- ½ chopped medium yellow onion
- 1 diced green bell pepper
- 1lb.can diced tomatoes with juices
- 1½ teaspoons ground cumin
- 1 tablespoon chilli powder
- 1 (6oz.) can low-Carbs tomato paste
- ⅓ cup water

Toppings:

- 1 cup sour cream
- ½ cup sliced green onions
- 2 tablespoons sliced jalapeños
- ½ cup shredded Cheddar cheese

Directions:

1. In a pot, add sausage and beef. Cook until browned. Break the clumps with a wooden spoon. Pat dry with paper towels. Reserve half of the meat for drippings.
2. Transfer the meat to a slow cooker. Add the reserved drippings, garlic, onion, bell pepper, tomatoes with juices, cumin, chilli powder, tomato paste, and water. Mix well to combine.
3. Put the slow cooker lid on, then cook for about 8 hours until the vegetables become soft.
4. Transfer them to serving plates. Top with sour cream, green onions, sliced jalapeños, and shredded cheese before serving.

Nutrition: Calories: 388 - Fat: 24.7g - Total Carbs: 10.6g - Fibre: 2.9g - Protein: 33.4g.

95. Basil-Rubbed Pork Chops

Preparation time: 15 minutes
Cooking time: 25 minutes
Servings: 4
Ingredients:

- 8oz. pork chops
- 1 lime, juiced
- ¼ cup fresh basil, chopped
- 1 garlic clove, minced
- Salt and freshly ground black pepper, to taste
- 1 tablespoon olive oil

Directions:

1. Place the pork chops in a baking tray and drizzle lime juice over them to coat. Rub the basil, garlic, salt and black pepper over the chops.
2. Cover the chops and let stand for about 30 minutes.
3. Meanwhile, preheat an outdoor grill on medium heat, and lightly grease its grate with olive oil.
4. Transfer the marinated pork chops to the grill and cook for 10 minutes per side until the internal temperature reaches 145°F.
5. Let cool for about 5 minutes before serving.

Nutrition: Calories: 512 - Fat: 28.5g - Total Carbs: 2.1g - Fibre: 0.2g - Protein: 58.4g.

96. Roast Beef and Mozzarella Plate

Preparation time: 5 minutes
Cooking time: 0 minutes
Servings: 2
Ingredients:

- 6 slices of roast beef
- ½oz. chopped lettuce
- 1 avocado, pitted
- 1 cup mozzarella cheese, cubed
- ½ cup mayonnaise
- ¼ tsp salt
- 1/8 tsp ground black pepper
- Avocado oil

Directions:

1. Scoop out flesh from avocado and divide it evenly between two plates.
2. Add slices of roast beef, lettuce, and cheese and then sprinkle with salt and black pepper.
3. Serve with avocado oil and mayonnaise.

Nutrition: Calories: 268 - Fat: 24.5g - Protein: 9.5g - Carbs: 1.5g - Fibre: 2g.

97. Beef Tenderloin Steaks Wrapped with Bacon

Preparation time: 10 minutes
Cooking time: 15 minutes
Servings: 4
Ingredients:

- 4oz. beef tenderloin steaks
- Sea salt and ground black pepper to taste
- 8 bacon slices
- 1 tablespoon extra-virgin olive oil

Directions:

1. Preheat the oven to 450°F and line the baking sheet with parchment paper.
2. Arrange the steaks on a flat surface. Sprinkle with salt and pepper.
3. Wrap each steak tightly at the edges with 2 bacon slices and use toothpicks to secure.
4. Heat the olive oil in a skillet over medium-high heat.
5. Pan sear each side of the steaks for about 4 minutes and transfer to the baking sheet.
6. Roast the steaks in the preheated oven for 6 minutes until they are well browned on both sides.
7. Transfer the steaks to a flat surface to cool for about 10 minutes.
8. Remove the toothpicks before serving.

Nutrition: Calories: 564 - Fat: 48.g - Total Carbs: 0g - Fibre: 0g - Protein: 27g.

98. Marinated Steak Sirloin Kabobs

Preparation time: 15 minutes
Cooking time: 10 minutes
Servings: 3
Ingredients:
Marinade:

- 1½ teaspoons paprika
- 1 teaspoon ground cumin
- 1 tablespoon chilli powder
- ½ teaspoon garlic powder
- ½ teaspoon salt
- Juice of 1 lime
- 2 tablespoons avocado oil

Kabobs:

- 1lb. boneless sirloin steak, sliced into 1-inch cubes
- 1 red bell pepper
- 1 green bell pepper
- ½ red onion, peeled and sliced in 1-inch pieces
- Sliced jalapeños, for garnish

Special equipment:

- bamboo skewers (about 10 inches), soaked for at least 30 minutes

Directions:

1. Put the steak in a Ziploc bag, then set aside.
2. Make the marinade: In a small bowl, mix the paprika, cumin, chilli, garlic, and salt, then mix well with a fork. Add the lime juice and avocado oil, then mix well. Transfer the mixture into the steak bag and seal tightly. Swing slowly to allow the pieces to coat evenly in the marinade. Transfer the bag into the refrigerator and chill for 45 minutes.
3. Preheat the grill to medium-high heat.
4. Deseed and remove membranes from the red and green bell peppers, then chop into 1-inch chunks.
5. Thread the marinated steak, onions, and peppers alternately onto the skewers.
6. Allow the kabobs to grill for 10 minutes or until browned.
7. Transfer to serving plates and garnish with the jalapeños before serving.

Nutrition: Calories: 428 - Fat: 28.9g - Total Carbs: 8.4g - Fibre: 3.0g - Protein: 33g.

99. Beef Mini Meatloaves with Bacon Wrappings

Preparation time: 10 minutes
Cooking time: 30 minutes
Servings: 8
Ingredients:

- 1lb. ground beef
- ⅓ cup nutritional yeast
- ¾ teaspoon ground gray sea salt
- ¼ cup low-Carbs tomato sauce
- 1 tablespoon prepared yellow mustard
- ¼ teaspoon ground black pepper
- 1oz. strips bacon

Directions:

1. Preheat the oven to 350°F.
2. In a bowl, add the beef, yeast, salt, tomato sauce, mustard, and pepper. Mix well with your hands.
3. Make the mini meatloaves: Scoop out 1 tablespoon portions and roll to form a cylinder. Repeat with the remaining mixture to make 8 cylinders. Wrap each of the cylinders with one strip of bacon. Transfer the wrapped cylinders to a cast-iron pan (loose ends of the bacon facing down) with a spacing of ½ inch between cylinders.
4. Bake in the preheated oven for about 30 minutes or until an instant-read thermometer inserted in the center registers 165°F.
5. Adjust the oven broiler to high. Allow the mini meatloaves to broil for 2 minutes until the bacon is crispy.
6. Transfer to a serving platter to cool before serving.

Nutrition: Calories: 295 - Fat: 21.2g - Total Carbs: 3.2g - Fibre: 1.0g - Protein: 21.9g.

100. Sloppy Joes

Preparation time: 15 minutes
Cooking time: 40 minutes
Servings: 8
Ingredients:

- ¼ cup plus 1½ teaspoons refined avocado oil
- 1 teaspoon cumin seeds
- 2 small, minced cloves garlic
- 1 minced piece fresh ginger root
- ¼ cup red onions, finely diced
- 1lb. ground beef
- 1⅔ cups low-Carbs tomato sauce
- 2 crushed whole dried chillies
- ¾ cup water
- 2 teaspoons curry powder
- ½ teaspoon paprika
- 1 teaspoon finely ground gray sea salt
- ⅓ cup raw macadamia nut halves
- 1 tablespoon apple cider vinegar
- ½ cup unsweetened coconut milk
- ¼ cup chopped fresh cilantro leaves, plus more for garnish
- Endives, leaves separated, plus more for garnish

Directions:

1. Make Sloppy Joes: Add ¼ cup oil, cumin seeds, garlic, ginger, and onions in a saucepan. Cook over medium heat for about 3 minutes until the onions are fragrant.
2. Add the beef to cook for about 8 minutes until it loses the pink color. Stir occasionally to break the beef into small clumps.
3. Add the tomato sauce, crushed chillies, water, curry powder, paprika, and salt and stir thoroughly to mix. Cover the lid partially to allow the steam to escape. Bring to a boil before adjusting the heat to medium-low to simmer for 25 minutes.
4. In a frying pan over medium-low heat, add the remaining oil and macadamia nuts. Roast for about 3 minutes until lightly golden. Toss constantly.
5. After 25 minutes of simmering, add the vinegar and coconut milk to the meat mixture. Adjust to medium-high heat and cook for about 5 minutes until thickened.
6. Add the cilantro and roasted nuts into the meat mixture. Stir well to mix.
7. Divide the endive leaves equally on 8 plates. Top with Sloppy Joes using a spoon.
8. Garnish the meal with extra cilantro and endives before serving.

Nutrition: Calories: 340 - Fat: 26.8g - Total Carbs: 8.1g - Fibre: 2.7g - Protein: 16.5g.

101. Curried Ground Sausage

Preparation time: 5 minutes
Cooking time: 15 minutes
Servings: 2
Ingredients:

- 7oz. sausage, crumbled
- 1 green onion, sliced
- 2.8oz. spinach
- 1oz. chicken bone broth
- 1oz. whipping cream
- 1 tbsp avocado oil
- ½ tsp garlic powder
- 1 tbsp curry powder
- ¼ cup of water

Directions:

1. Take a medium saucepan, place it over medium heat, add ½ tbsp oil and when hot, add ground sausage and cook for 4 to 5 minutes until cooked.
2. When done, transfer sausage to a bowl, add remaining oil and when hot, add green onion, sprinkle with garlic powder and cook for 2 minutes until sauté.
3. Sprinkle with curry powder, continue cooking for 30 seconds until fragrant, pour in chicken broth and water, add sausage and spinach, stir until mixed and simmer for 5 minutes until thickened slightly.
4. Taste to adjust seasoning, stir in cream and then remove the pan from heat.
5. Serve.

Nutrition: Calories: 435 - Fat: 42g - Protein: 12g Carbs:1.4g - Fibre: 0.8g.

102. Cheese, Olives and Sausage Casserole

Preparation time: 10 minutes
Cooking time: 15 minutes
Servings: 3
Ingredients:
- 10oz. sausage
- 3oz green olives, sliced
- 2 eggs
- 3oz. coconut milk, unsweetened
- 1 tbsp grated cheddar cheese

Seasoning:
- ¼ tsp ground black pepper
- 1/3 tsp salt
- 1/3 tsp mustard powder

Directions:
1. Take a medium skillet pan, place it over medium heat and when hot, add sausage, crumble it and cook for 5 minutes until cooked.
2. Meanwhile, crack eggs in a medium bowl, add milk, salt, black pepper, and mustard and whisk until blended.
3. When sausage had cooked, add sausage mixture into the eggs, add onion and olives, 2 tbsp cheese, and then stir until mixed.
4. Then spoon the mixture into a casserole dish, cover with a lid and let it refrigerate for 1 hour until chilled.
5. When ready to bake, turn on the oven, then set it to 350°F and let it preheat.
6. Sprinkle cheese on the top casserole and then bake it for 10 minutes until cheese has melted.
7. Serve.

Nutrition: Calories: 351- Fat:31g - Protein: 15.5g - Carbs: 1.7g - Fibre: 0.9g.

103. Portobello Mushrooms with Sausage and Cheese

Preparation time: 10 minutes
Cooking time: 20 minutes
Servings: 2
Ingredients:
- 4 portobello mushroom caps
- 7oz. sausage
- 1 tbsp melted butter, unsalted
- 1 tbsp grated parmesan cheese
- 1/8 tsp garlic powder
- 1/8 tsp red chilli powder
- ¼ tsp salt
- Avocado oil

Directions:
1. Turn on the oven, then set it to 425°F and let it preheat.
2. Meanwhile, remove the stems from mushroom caps, chop them and then brush the caps with butter inside-out.
3. Take a frying pan, place it over medium heat, add oil and when hot, add sausage, crumble it, sprinkle with garlic powder and then cook for 5 minutes until cooked.
4. Stir in mushroom stems, season with salt and black pepper, continue cooking for 3 minutes until cooked and then remove the pan from heat.
5. Distribute sausage-mushroom mixture into mushroom caps, sprinkle cheese, and red chilli powder on top and then bake for 10 to 12 minutes until mushroom caps have turned tender and cooked. Serve.

Nutrition: Calorie: 310 - Fat: 26g -Protein: 10.7g Carbs: 6.6g - Fibre:1.1g.

104. Smoked Sausage and Cauliflower Fried Rice

Preparation time: 15 minutes
Cooking time: 15 minutes.
Servings: 4
Ingredients:

- 3 tablespoons vegetable oil, divided
- 1 package (12oz.) of smoked sausage cut to 1/2 inch
- 4 cups small broccoli florets
- 1 medium red bell pepper, cut into strips
- 2 large eggs, lightly beaten
- 1 (12oz.) package frozen riced cauliflower
- ¼ cup reduced-sodium soy sauce
- 1 tablespoon toasted sesame oil
- ½ teaspoon granulated sugar
- ½ teaspoon black pepper
- 2 tablespoons chopped cilantro

Directions:

1. In a large nonstick skillet, heat 1 tablespoon of the oil over medium-high. Add sausage; cook about 3 minutes, stirring occasionally, until lightly browned. Add broccoli and bell pepper; cook 5-6 minutes, stirring occasionally, until broccoli is bright green and slightly tender. Remove mixture to a plate.
2. Wipe skillet clean-careful, may be hot-reduce heat to medium, and add 1 tablespoon oil. Add eggs. Cook 2-3 minutes until set, stirring once or twice. Transfer to a cutting board and cut into 1/2-inch pieces.
3. Return skillet to stove over medium-high. Add remaining 1 tablespoon oil. Add cauliflower; cook, undisturbed, until softened and lightly toasted, about 4 minutes. Remove from heat. Stir in soy sauce, sesame oil, sugar, pepper, sausage mixture, and egg. Divide among plates and top with cilantro.

Nutrition: Calories: 498 - Fat: 40.6g - Protein: 19.3g - Carbs: 18.4g.

105. Cheesy Sausage and Egg Bake

Preparation time: 5 minutes
Cooking time: 18 minutes
Servings: 2
Ingredients:

- 7.5oz. sausage
- 1 egg
- 1 tbsp grated cheddar cheese
- 1 ½ tbsp grated mozzarella cheese
- 1 ½ tbsp grated parmesan cheese
- ¼ tsp salt
- 1/8 tsp ground black pepper
- Avocado oil

Directions:

1. Turn on the oven, then set it to 375°F and let it preheat.
2. Meanwhile, take a medium skillet pan, place it over medium heat, add oil and when hot, add sausage and cook for 5 minutes until cooked.
3. Meanwhile, crack the egg in a medium bowl, add salt, black pepper, and cheeses, reserving 1 tbsp cheddar cheese and whisk until mixed.
4. When the sausage has cooked, transfer it to the bowl containing egg batter and stir until combined.
5. Take a baking pan, grease it with oil, pour in sausage mixture, sprinkle remaining cheddar cheese in the top, and then bake for 10 to 12 minutes until cooked.
6. When done, let sausage cool for 5 minutes, then cut it into squares and then serve.

Nutrition: Calories: 439 - Fat: 39g - Protein: 19.7g - Carbs: 2.2g - Fibre: 0g.

106. Sausage and Marinara Casserole

Preparation time: 5 minutes
Cooking time: 12 minutes
Servings: 2
Ingredients:

- 5.5oz. chorizo
- 5.5oz. sausage
- 1 tbsp avocado oil
- 2 cup marinara sauce
- 1 tbsp grated cheddar cheese
- ¼ tsp salt
- 1/8 tsp ground black pepper
- ¼ tsp dried thyme

Directions:

1. Take a medium skillet pan, place it over medium heat, add oil and when hot, add chorizo and sausage and cook for 4 to 5 minutes until meat is no longer pink.
2. Add the marinara sauce into the pan, stir in salt, black pepper, and thyme, cook for 1 minute until hot and then transfer meat mixture into a casserole dish.
3. Sprinkle cheese over the top of casserole and then bake for 7 minutes until thoroughly cooked. Serve.

Nutrition: Calories: 485 - Fat: 44.4g - Protein: 15.6g - Carbs: 3.7g - Fibre:1.1g.

107. Double Cheese Meatloaf

Preparation time: 10 minutes
Cooking time: 20 minutes
Servings: 2
Ingredients:

- 2 slices of bacon, chopped, cooked
- 8oz of minced sausage
- 1 tbsp grated mozzarella cheese
- 1 tbsp grated cheddar cheese
- 1/3 tsp salt
- 1/4 tsp ground black pepper
- 1 tsp dried parsley
- 1 tbsp marinara sauce
- 1 egg

Directions:

1. Turn on the oven, then set it to 375°F and let it preheat.

2. Meanwhile, take a medium bowl, place all the ingredients in it except for marinara and stir until well combined.
3. Spoon the mixture into a mini loaf pan, top with marinara, and then bake for 20 to 25 minutes until cooked through and done.
4. When done, let meatloaf cool for 5 minutes, then cut it into slices and then serve.

Nutrition: Calories: 578 - Fat:50.6g - Protein:27.4g - Carbs: 2.6g - Fibre: 0.3g.

108. Spinach Sausage Ball Pasta

Preparation time: 10 minutes
Cooking time: 12 minutes
Servings: 2
Ingredients:

- 1lb. cabbage, shredded
- 1/2lb. sausage
- 5oz. spinach, chopped
- 1 tbsp grated parmesan cheese
- 1 tbsp marinara sauce
- 1/3 tsp salt
- ¼ tsp ground black pepper
- Avocado oil

Directions:

1. Take a medium bowl, place sausage in it, add spinach and cheese in it, season with 1/3 tsp salt and black pepper, stir until well combined, and then shape the mixture into balls.
2. Take a medium skillet pan, place it over medium heat, add 1 tbsp oil and when hot, add meatballs and cook for 3 to 4 minutes per side until cooked and nicely golden brown.
3. When transfer meatballs to a plate, add remaining oil into the pan and, when hot, add cabbage and then cook for 3 minutes until tender-crisp.
4. Return meatballs into the pan, add marinara sauce, toss until well mixed and cook for 1 minute until hot. Serve.

Nutrition: Calories: 505 - Fat: 42g - Protein: 18.7g - Carbs: 6.5g - Fibre: 6g.

109. Beef with Cabbage Noodles

Preparation time: 5 minutes
Cooking time: 18 minutes
Servings: 2
Ingredients:
- 2lb. ground beef
- 2 cup chopped cabbage
- 24oz. tomato sauce
- ½ tsp minced garlic
- ½ cup of water
- ½ tbsp coconut oil
- ½ tsp salt
- ¼ tsp Italian seasoning
- 1/8 tsp dried basil

Directions:
1. Take a skillet pan, place it over medium heat, add oil and when hot, add beef and cook for 5 minutes until nicely browned.
2. Meanwhile, prepare the cabbage and for it, slice the cabbage into thin shred.
3. When the beef has cooked, add garlic, season with salt, basil, and Italian seasoning, stir well and continue cooking for 3 minutes until beef has thoroughly cooked.
4. Pour in tomato sauce and water, stir well and bring the mixture to boil.
5. Then reduce heat to medium-low level, add cabbage, stir well until well mixed and simmer for 3 to 5 minutes until cabbage is softened, covering the pan.
6. Uncover the pan and continue simmering the beef until most of the cooking liquid has evaporated.
7. Serve.

Nutrition: Calories:188.5 - Fat: 12.5g - Protein: 15.5g - Fibre: 1g - Carbs: 2.5g.

110. Garlic Herb Beef Roast

Preparation time: 5 minutes
Cooking time: 10 minutes
Servings: 2
Ingredients:
- 6 slices of beef roast
- ½ tsp garlic powder
- 1/3 tsp dried thyme
- ¼ tsp dried rosemary
- 1 tbsp butter, unsalted
- 1/3 tsp salt
- 1/4 tsp ground black pepper

Directions:
1. Prepare the spice mix and for this, take a small bowl, place garlic powder, thyme, rosemary, salt, and black pepper and then stir until mixed.
2. Sprinkle spices mix on the beef roast.
3. Take a medium skillet pan, place it over medium heat, add butter and when it melts, add beef roast and then cook for 5 to 8 minutes until golden brown and cooked.
4. Serve.

Nutrition: Calories: 140 - Fat: 12.7g - Protein: 5.5g - Carbs: 0.1g - Fibre: 0.2g.

111. Beef and Vegetable Skillet

Preparation time: 5 minutes
Cooking time: 15 minutes
Servings: 2
Ingredients:
- 3oz. spinach, chopped
- ½ pound ground beef
- 1 slices of bacon, diced
- 3oz. chopped asparagus
- 1 tbsp coconut oil
- 1 tsp dried thyme
- 2/3 tsp salt
- ½ tsp ground black pepper

Directions:
1. Take a skillet pan, place it over medium heat, add oil and when hot, add beef and bacon and cook for 5 to 7 minutes until slightly browned.
2. Then add asparagus and spinach, sprinkle with thyme, stir well and cook for 7 to 10 minutes until thoroughly cooked.
3. Season skillet with salt and black pepper and serve.

Nutrition: Calories: 332.5 - Fat: 26g - Protein: 23.5g - Carbs:1.5g - Fibre: 1g.

112. Sprouts Stir-fry with Kale, Broccoli, and Beef

Preparation time: 5 minutes
Cooking time: 8 minutes
Servings: 2
Ingredients:
- 1lb.slices of beef roast, chopped
- 1/2lb. brussels sprouts, halved
- 1 cup broccoli florets
- 1cup kale
- 1 ½ tbsp butter, unsalted
- 1/8 tsp red pepper flakes

Seasoning:
- ¼ tsp garlic powder
- ¼ tsp salt
- 1/8 tsp ground black pepper

Directions:
1. Take a medium skillet pan, place it over medium heat, add ¾ tbsp butter and when it melts, add broccoli florets and sprouts, sprinkle with garlic powder, and cook for 2 minutes.
2. Season vegetables with salt and red pepper flakes, add chopped beef, stir until mixed and continue cooking for 3 minutes until browned on one side.
3. Then add kale along with remaining butter, flip the vegetables and cook for 2 minutes until kale leaves wilts.
4. Serve.

Nutrition: Calories: 125 - Fat: 9.4g - Protein: 4.8g - Carbs: 1.7g - Fibre: 2.6g.

113. Beef, Pepper and Green Beans Stir-fry

Preparation time: 5 minutes
Cooking time: 18 minutes
Servings: 2
Ingredients:
- ½lb. ground beef
- 1 chopped green bell pepper
- ½ lb. green beans
- 1 tbsp grated cheddar cheese
- ½ tsp salt
- ¼ tsp ground black pepper
- ¼ tsp paprika

Directions:
1. Take a skillet pan, place it over medium heat, add ground beef and cook for 4 minutes until slightly browned.
2. Then add bell pepper and green beans, season with salt, paprika, and black pepper, stir well and continue cooking for 7 to 10 minutes until beef and vegetables have cooked through.
3. Sprinkle cheddar cheese on top, then transfer pan under the broiler and cook for 2 minutes until cheese has melted and the top is golden brown. Serve.

Nutrition: Calories: 282.5 - Fat: 17.6g - Protein: 26g - Carbs: 3g - Fibre: 2.1g.

114. Cheesy Meatloaf

Preparation time: 5 minutes
Cooking time: 4 minutes
Servings: 2
Ingredients:
- ½lb. ground turkey
- 1 egg
- 1 tbsp grated mozzarella cheese
- ¼ tsp Italian seasoning
- ½ tbsp soy sauce
- ¼ tsp salt
- 1/8 tsp ground black pepper

Directions:
1. Take a bowl, place all the ingredients in it, and stir until mixed.
2. Take a heatproof mug, spoon in prepared mixture and microwave for 3 minutes at high heat setting until cooked.
3. When done, let meatloaf rest in the mug for 1 minute, then take it out, cut it into two slices and serve.

Nutrition: Calories: 196.5 - Fat: 13.5g - Protein: 18.7g - Fibre: 0g - Carbs:18.7g.

115.   Roast Beef and Vegetable Plate

Preparation time: 10 minutes
Cooking time: 10 minutes
Servings: 2
Ingredients:
- 1 scallion, chopped in large pieces
- 1 ½ tbsp coconut oil
- 4 thin slices of roast beef
- 7oz. cauliflower and broccoli mix
- 1 tbsp butter, unsalted
- 1/2 tsp salt
- 1/3 tsp ground black pepper
- 1 tsp dried parsley

Directions:
1. Turn on the oven, then set it to 400°F, and let it preheat.
2. Take a baking sheet, grease it with oil, place slices of roast beef on one side, and top with butter.
3. Take a separate bowl, add cauliflower and broccoli mix, add scallions, drizzle with oil, season with remaining salt and black pepper, toss until coated and then spread vegetables on the empty side of the baking sheet.
4. Bake for 5 to 7 minutes until beef is nicely browned and vegetables are tender-crisp, tossing halfway.
5. Distribute beef and vegetables between two plates and then serve.

Nutrition: Calories: 313 -Fat: 26g - Protein: 15.6g - Carbs: 2.8g - Fibre: 1.9g.

116.   Grilled Moroccan-Spiced Rack of Lamb

Preparation Time: 15 minutes
Cooking Time: 30-35 minutes
Servings: 4
Ingredients:
For the spice blend:
- ⅓ cup finely chopped fresh cilantro
- ⅓ cup finely chopped fresh parsley
- ¼ cup freshly squeezed lemon juice of about 2 lemons
- 1 tbsp. extra virgin olive oil
- 1 tbsp. freshly sliced garlic, about 3 medium-sized teeth

For the spice and lamb sauce:
- 1 tbsp. bell pepper
- 1 tbsp. kosher salt
- 1 tsp ground cumin
- 1 tsp ground coriander
- 1 tsp freshly ground black pepper
- ½ tsp cinnamon
- ¼ tsp cayenne pepper
- lamb chops, 7-10 ribs, sliced everything but a thin layer of fat, about 1 ½ lb. each
- 1 tbsp. dijon mustard

Directions:
1. For the spice mix: combine the coriander, parsley, lemon juice, olive oil, and garlic in a medium bowl. Set aside.
2. For the Rub Spice: combine the pepper, salt, cumin, coriander, black pepper, cinnamon, and cayenne pepper in a small bowl. Season the lamb chops with the spice blend.
3. Light a fireplace full of coals. When all the charcoal is lit and covered with gray ash, pour and place the charcoal on 1 side of the charcoal grate. Place the grill in its place, cover the grill, and let it preheat for 5 minutes. Clean and grease the grill. Bring the lamb chops on the hot side of the restaurant, fat side down, and cook until golden, 3 to 5 minutes. Place the lamb on a cutting board.
4. Brush a thin layer of mustard on the thick side of each rack of lamb. Gently squeeze the mixture of herbs and lemon into the mustard in each box and spread evenly.
5. Put the grills back in the grill, the fat in place closed, but not directly above, the coals. Continue cooking until an immediately readable thermometer registers 130°F when placed at the bottom of the rack for 15 to 25 min. Remove from grill, leave uncovered for 10 min Cut between ribs in chops, and serve immediately.

Nutrition: Calories: 374 - Protein: 48g - Fat: 19.1g - Carbs: 3.36g.

117. Lamb Burgers with Tzatziki

Preparation Time: 10 minutes
Cooking Time: 20 minutes
Servings: 4
Ingredients:

- 1lb. of grass-fed lamb
- ¼ cup chives finely chopped green onion or red onion if desired
- 1 tbsp. chopped fresh dill
- ½ tsp dried oregano or about 1 tbsp. freshly chopped
- 1 tbsp. finely chopped fresh mint
- A pinch of chopped red pepper
- Fine-grained sea salt
- 1 tbsp. water
- 1 tsp olive oil to grease the pan

For the tzatziki:

- 1 can coconut milk with all the cooled fat and 1 tbsp. the discarded liquid portion
- 2 cloves of garlic
- 1 peeled cucumber without seeds, roughly sliced
- 1 tbsp. freshly squeezed lemon juice
- 1 tbsp. chopped fresh dill
- 3/4 tsp fine grain sea salt
- Black pepper to taste

Directions:

1. To make the tzatziki:
2. Place the garlic, cucumber, and lemon juice in the food processor and press until finely chopped. Add the coconut cream, dill, salt, and pepper, and mix until well blended.
3. Put it in a jar with a lid and keep it in the refrigerator until it is served. The flavors become more intense over time when they cool in the fridge.
4. For burgers:
5. Thoroughly mix the ground lamb in a bowl with the chives or red onion, dill, oregano, mint, red pepper, and water.
6. Sprinkle the mixture with fine-grained sea salt and form 4 patties of the same size.
7. Heat a large cast-iron skillet over medium heat and brush with a small amount of olive oil. Lightly sprinkle the pan with fine-grain sea salt.
8. Bring the patties into the pan and cook on each side for about 4 min, adjusting the heat to prevent the outside from becoming too brown. Alternatively, you can grill the burgers.
9. Remove from the pan and cover with tzatziki sauce.

Nutrition: Calories: 363 - Protein: 35.33g - Fat: 22g - Carbs: 6.83g.

Chapter 11. Poultry

118.   Parmesan Baked Chicken

Preparation time: 5 minutes
Cooking time: 20 minutes
Servings: 2
Ingredients:
- 2 tablespoons ghee
- 2 boneless skinless chicken breasts
- Pink Himalayan salt
- Freshly ground black pepper
- ½ cup mayonnaise
- ¼ cup grated Parmesan cheese
- 1 tablespoon dried Italian seasoning
- ¼ cup crushed pork rinds

Directions:
1. Preheat the oven to 425°F. Choose a baking dish that is large enough to hold both chicken breasts and coat it with the ghee.
2. Pat dry the chicken breasts with a paper towel, season with pink Himalayan salt and pepper, and place in the prepared baking dish.
3. In a small bowl, mix to combine the mayonnaise, Parmesan cheese, and Italian seasoning.
4. Slather the mayonnaise mixture evenly over the chicken breasts, and sprinkle the crushed pork rinds on top of the mayonnaise mixture.
5. Bake until the topping is browned, about 20 minutes, and serve.

Nutrition: Calories: 850 - Fat: 67g - Carbs: 2g - Protein: 60g - Fibre: 0g.

119.   Garlic-Parmesan Chicken Wings

Preparation time: 10 minutes
Cooking time: 3 hours
Servings:2
Ingredients:
- 1 small stick of butter
- Garlic cloves, minced
- 1 tablespoon dried Italian seasoning
- ¼ cup grated Parmesan cheese, plus ½ cup
- Pink Himalayan salt
- Freshly ground black pepper
- 1lb. chicken wings

Directions:
1. With the crock insert in place, preheat the slow cooker to high. Line a baking sheet with aluminum foil or a silicone baking mat.
2. Put the butter, garlic, Italian seasoning, and ¼ cup of Parmesan cheese in the slow cooker, and season with pink Himalayan salt and pepper. Allow the butter to melt and stir the ingredients until well mixed.
3. Add the chicken wings and stir until coated with the butter mixture.
4. Cover the slow cooker and cook for 2 hours and 45 minutes.
5. Preheat the broiler.
6. Transfer the wings to the prepared baking sheet, sprinkle the remaining ½ cup of Parmesan cheese over the wings, and cook under the broiler until crispy, about 5 minutes.
7. Serve hot.

Nutrition: Calories: 738 - Fat: 66g - Carbs: 4g - Protein: 39g - Fibre: 0g.

120.   Chicken Skewers with Peanut Sauce

Preparation time: 10 minutes, plus 1 hour to marinate
Cooking time: 15 minutes
Servings: 2
Ingredients:

- 1 chicken breast, cut into chunks
- 3 tablespoons soy sauce (or coconut aminos), divided
- ½ teaspoon Sriracha sauce, plus ¼ teaspoon
- 3 teaspoons of toasted sesame oil, divided
- Ghee, for oiling
- 1 teaspoon of peanut butter
- Pink Himalayan salt
- Freshly ground black pepper

Directions:

1. In a large zip-up bag, combine the chicken pieces with 2 tablespoons of soy sauce, ½ teaspoon of Sriracha sauce and 2 teaspoons of sesame oil. Close the bag and let the chicken marinate for about an hour in the refrigerator or overnight.
2. If you are using 8-inch wooden skewers, soak them in water for 30 minutes before use.
3. Preheat the grill over low heat (or a large skillet). Oil with ghee.
4. Place the chicken pieces on the skewers.
5. Cook the skewers over low heat for 10-15 minutes, turning them halfway.
6. Meanwhile, stir in the peanut sauce. Mix the remaining 1 tablespoon of soy sauce, ¼ teaspoon of Sriracha sauce, 1 teaspoon of sesame oil and peanut butter. Season with pink Himalayan salt and pepper.
7. Serve the chicken skewers with a saucer of peanut sauce.

Nutrition: Calories: 586 - Fat: 29g - Carbs: 5g - Protein: 75g - Fibre: 1g.

121.   Braised Chicken Thighs with Kalamata Olives

Preparation time: 10 minutes
Cooking time: 40 minutes
Servings: 2
Ingredients:

- 4 chicken thighs, skin on
- Pink Himalayan salt
- Freshly ground black pepper
- 2 tablespoons ghee
- ½ cup chicken broth
- 1 lemon, ½ sliced and ½ juiced
- ½ cup pitted Kalamata olives
- Butter

Directions:

1. Preheat the oven to 370°F.
2. Pat the chicken thighs dry with paper towels, and season with pink Himalayan salt and pepper.
3. In a medium oven-safe skillet or high-sided baking dish over medium-high heat, melt the ghee. When the ghee has melted and is hot, add the chicken thighs, skin-side down, and leave them for about 8 minutes, or until the skin is brown and crispy.
4. Flip the chicken and cook for 2 minutes on the second side. Around the chicken thighs, pour in the chicken broth, and add the lemon slices, lemon juice, and olives.
5. Bake in the oven for about 30 minutes, until the chicken is cooked through.
6. Add the butter to the broth mixture.
7. Divide the chicken and olives between two plates and serve.

Nutrition: Calories: 567 - Fat: 47g - Carbs: 2g - Protein: 33g - Fibre: 2g.

122.   Buttery Garlic Chicken

Preparation time: 5 minutes
Cooking time: 40 minutes
Servings: 2
Ingredients:

- 2 tablespoons ghee, melted
- 2 boneless skinless chicken breasts
- Pink Himalayan salt
- Freshly ground black pepper
- 1 tablespoon dried Italian seasoning
- 1 tablespoons butter
- 1 garlic clove, minced
- ¼ cup grated Parmesan cheese

Directions:

1. Preheat the oven to 375°F. Choose a baking dish that is large enough to hold both chicken breasts and coat it with the ghee.
2. Pat dry the chicken breasts and season with pink Himalayan salt, pepper, and Italian seasoning. Place the chicken in the baking dish.
3. In a medium skillet over medium heat, melt the butter. Add the minced garlic and cook for about 5 minutes. You want the garlic very lightly browned but not burned.
4. Remove the butter-garlic mixture from the heat and pour it over the chicken breasts.
5. Roast the chicken in the oven for 30 to 35 minutes, until cooked through. Sprinkle some of the Parmesan cheese on top of each chicken breast. Let the chicken rest in the baking dish for 5 minutes.
6. Divide the chicken between two plates, spoon the butter sauce over the chicken, and serve.

Nutrition: Calories: 642 - Fat: 45g - Carbs: 2g - Protein: 57g - Fibre: 0g.

123.   Cheesy Bacon and Broccoli Chicken

Preparation time: 10 minutes
Cooking time: 1 hour
Servings: 2
Ingredients:

- 2 tablespoons ghee
- 2 boneless skinless chicken breasts
- Pink Himalayan salt
- Freshly ground black pepper
- 4 bacon slices
- 3.5oz. cream cheese, at room temperature
- 2 cups frozen broccoli florets, thawed
- ½ cup shredded Cheddar cheese

Directions:

1. Preheat the oven to 375°F.
2. Choose a baking dish that is large enough to hold both chicken breasts and coat it with the ghee.
3. Pat dry the chicken breasts with a paper towel, and season with pink Himalayan salt and pepper.
4. Place the chicken breasts and the bacon slices in the baking dish, and bake for 25 minutes.
5. Transfer the chicken to a cutting board and use two forks to shred it. Season it again with pink Himalayan salt and pepper.
6. Place the bacon on a paper towel–lined plate to crisp up, and then crumble it.
7. In a medium bowl, mix to combine the cream cheese, shredded chicken, broccoli, and half of the bacon crumbles. Transfer the chicken mixture to the baking dish, and top with the Cheddar and the remaining half of the bacon crumbles.
8. Bake until the cheese is bubbling and browned, about 35 minutes, and serve.

Nutrition: Calories: 935 - Fat: 66g - Carbs: 8g - Protein: 75g - Fibre: 3g.

124.   Crunchy Chicken Milanese

Preparation time: 10 minutes
Cooking time: 10 minutes
Servings: 2
Ingredients:

- 2 boneless skinless chicken breasts
- ½ cup coconut flour
- 1 teaspoon ground cayenne pepper
- Pink Himalayan salt
- Freshly ground black pepper
- 1 egg, lightly beaten
- ½ cup crushed pork rinds
- 2 tablespoons olive oil

Directions:

1. Pound the chicken breasts with a heavy mallet until they are about ½ inch thick. (If you don't have a kitchen mallet, you can use the thick rim of a heavy plate.)
2. Prepare two separate prep plates and one small, shallow bowl:
3. On plate 1, put the coconut flour, cayenne pepper, pink Himalayan salt, and pepper. Mix together.
4. Crack the egg into the small bowl, and lightly beat it with a fork or whisk.
5. On plate 2, put the crushed pork rinds.
6. In a large skillet over medium-high heat, heat the olive oil.
7. Dredge 1 chicken breast on both sides in the coconut-flour mixture. Dip the chicken into the egg, and coat both sides. Dredge the chicken in the pork-rind mixture, pressing the pork rinds into the chicken so they stick. Place the coated chicken in the hot skillet and repeat with the other chicken breast.
8. Cook the chicken for 3 to 5 minutes on each side, until brown, crispy, and cooked through, and serve.

Nutrition: Calories: 604 - Fat: 29g - Carbs: 7g - Protein: 65g - Fibre: 10g.

125.   Egg Butter

Preparation time: 5 minutes
Cooking time: 0 minutes
Servings: 2
Ingredients:

- 3 large eggs, hard-boiled
- 3oz. unsalted butter
- ½ tsp dried oregano
- ½ tsp dried basil
- 2 leaves of iceberg lettuce

Seasoning:

- ½ tsp of sea salt
- ¼ tsp ground black pepper

Directions:

1. Peel the eggs, then chop them finely and place in a medium bowl.
2. Add remaining ingredients and stir well.
3. Serve egg butter wrapped in a lettuce leaf.

Nutrition: Calories: 159 - Fat: 16.5g - Protein: 3g Carbs: 0.2g - Fibre: 0g.

126.   Turkey and Potatoes with Buffalo Sauce

Preparation Time: 10 minutes
Cooking Time: 20 minutes
Servings: 2
Ingredients:

- Olive oil
- 1 tbsp. buffalo sauce
- 1 lb. sweet potatoes, cut into cubes
- 1 lb. turkey breast, cut into pieces
- ½ tsp garlic powder
- 1 onion, diced
- ½ cup water

Directions:

1. Heat 1 tbsp. Of olive oil. Stir-fry onion in hot oil for about 3 minutes. Add the other ingredients. Seal the lid, set to Pressure Cook mode for 15-20 minutes at high pressure.
2. When cooking is over, do a quick pressure release by turning the valve to an "open" position.

Nutrition: Calories: 377 - Carbs: 32g - Fat: 9g - Protein: 14g.

127. Delightful Teriyaki Chicken Under Pressure

Preparation Time: 15 minutes
Cooking Time: 20 minutes
Servings: 6
Ingredients:

- 1/2 cup of low sodium soy sauce
- 1/3 cup granulated sugar
- 1/3 cup water
- 2 tablespoons mirin
- 3 cloves garlic, chopped
- 1inch fresh ginger, peeled and grated
- 2 pounds boneless, skinless chicken thighs
- 1 tablespoon cornstarch
- 1 tablespoon water

Directions:

1. Select Sauté on Normal on pressure cooker. Stir soy sauce, sugar, water, mirin, garlic, and ginger together in the inner steel pot of pressure cooker until sugar has dissolved, 3 to 4 minutes; add chicken and turn to coat. Press Cancel.
2. Lock pressure cooker lid in place and set steam vent to Sealing. Select Pressure Cook (Manual) and cook for 12 minutes on /High Pressure. Turn steam vent to Venting to Quick Release the pressure. Press Cancel.
3. Transfer chicken to a cutting board; cut into ¼-inch-thick slices. Leave sauce in the pressure cooker.
4. Select Sauté on Normal.
5. Dissolve cornstarch into water in a small bowl, stirring with a fork until smooth; stir into sauce in the pot and cook, stirring often, until very thick and syrupy, 2 to 3 minutes.
6. Serve chicken over rice with sauce. Garnish with green onions and sesame seeds.

Nutrition: Calories: 342 - Carbs: 18g - Fat: 13g - Protein: 39g.

128. Shredded Chicken in a Lettuce Wrap

Preparation time: 5 minutes
Cooking time: 15 minutes
Servings: 2
Ingredients:

- 2 leaves of iceberg lettuce
- 1 large chicken thigh
- 1 tbsp shredded cheddar cheese
- 2 cups hot water
- 1 tbsp tomato sauce

Seasoning:

- 1 tbsp soy sauce
- 1 tbsp red chilli powder
- ¾ tsp salt
- ½ tsp cracked black pepper

Directions:

1. Turn on the instant pot, place chicken thighs in it, and add remaining ingredients except for lettuce.
2. Stir until just mixed, shut the instant pot with a lid and cook for 15 minutes at high pressure and when done, release the pressure naturally.
3. Then open the instant pot, transfer chicken to a cutting board and shred with two forks.
4. Evenly divide the chicken between two lettuce leaves, and drizzle with some of the cooking liquid, reserving the remaining cooking liquid for later use as chicken broth. Serve

Nutrition: Calories: 143.5 - Fat: 1.4g - Protein: 21.7g - Fibre: 0.7g - Carbs: 3.4g.

129.   Intermittent Chicken Enchiladas

Preparation Time: 10 minutes
Cooking Time: 25 minutes
Servings: 6
Ingredients:
- 2 cups gluten-free enchilada sauce
- 1 tablespoon avocado oil
- Garlic (minced)
- 2 cups shredded chicken (cooked)
- ¼ cup chicken broth
- ¼ cup fresh cilantro (chopped)
- 1 cup rice

Assembly
- Coconut tortillas
- 3/4 cup Colby jack cheese (shredded)
- ¼ cup green onions (chopped)

Direction:
1. Warm oil at medium to high heat in a large pan. Add the chopped garlic and cook until fragrant for about a minute.
2. Add the rice, chicken, 1 cup of enchilada sauce (half of the total), chicken broth and cilantro. Simmer for 5 minutes. In the meantime, heat the oven to 375°F. Grease a 9x13 baking dish.
3. In the center of each tortilla, place the chicken and rice mixture. Roll up and place seam side down in the baking dish.
4. Pour the remaining cup enchilada sauce over the enchiladas. Sprinkle with shredded cheese.
5. Bake for 8 to 10 minutes Sprinkle with green onions.

Nutrition: Calories: 349 - Fat: 19g - Carbs: 9g - Protein: 31g.

130.   Cider Chicken

Preparation time: 10 minutes
Cooking time: 18 minutes
Servings: 2
Ingredients:
- 2 chicken thighs
- ¼ cup apple cider vinegar
- 1 tsp liquid stevia

Seasoning:
- ½ tbsp coconut oil
- 1/3 tsp salt
- ¼ tsp ground black pepper

Directions:
1. Turn on the oven, then set it to 450°F and let it preheat.
2. Meanwhile, place chicken in a bowl, drizzle with oil and then season with salt and black pepper
3. Take a baking sheet, place prepared chicken thighs on it, and bake for 10 to 15 minutes or until its internal temperature reaches 175°F.
4. In the meantime, take a small saucepan, place it over medium heat, pour in vinegar, stir in stevia and bring the mixture to boil.
5. Then switch heat to the low level and simmer sauce for 3 to 5 minutes until reduced by half, set aside until required.
6. When the chicken has roasted, brush it generously with prepared cider sauce, then turn on the broiler and bake the chicken for 3 minutes until golden brown. Serve.

Nutrition: Calories: 182.5 - Fat: 107.5g - Protein: 15.5g - Fibre: 0g - Carbs: 2.5g.

131. Exquisite Pear and Onion Goose

Preparation Time: 15 minutes
Cooking Time: 20 minutes
Servings: 8
Ingredients:

- 2 ½ cups chicken broth
- 1 tbsp. of butter
- ½ cup slice onions
- 1 ½ pounds goose, chopped into large pieces
- 1 tbsp. balsamic vinegar
- 1 tsp cayenne pepper
- Pears, peeled and sliced
- ¼ tsp garlic powder
- ½ tsp of pepper

Directions:

1. Melt the butter on sauté. Add the goose and cook until it becomes golden on all sides. Transfer to a plate. Add the onions and cook for 3 minutes. Return the goose to the cooker.
2. Add the rest of the ingredients, stir well to combine and seal the lid. Select Pressure Cook (Manual) mode and set the timer to 16 minutes at High Pressure. Do a quick pressure release. Serve and enjoy!

Nutrition: Calories: 313 - Carbs: 14g - Fat: 8g - Protein: 38g.

132. Bacon-Wrapped Chicken with Cheddar Cheese

Preparation Time: 10 minutes
Cooking Time: 30 minutes
Servings: 4
Ingredients:

- 4 chicken breasts
- Cheddar cheese
- 4 slices of smoked bacon
- Pepper to taste
- Honey (optional)
- Whole grain mustard (optional)

Directions:

1. Preheat the oven to 350°F
2. Make a cut about 2cm deep in the chicken breast to about two thirds of the way into the flesh, cutting at an angle from the top along the breast. Fill with the cheese.
3. Slice the bacon into three strips lengthways. Wrap this around the chicken and tuck under the breast.
4. Warm a little oil in a frying pan over a medium heat then add the chicken. Season with pepper and cook for a few minutes until browned. Turn over and brown the other side, seasoning again with pepper. Remove from the frying pan and place on a baking tray.
5. Bake in the preheated oven until the chicken is no longer pink in the centre and the cheese has melted, about 20 minutes. Remove from the oven. Add a drizzle of honey and a good dollop of whole grain mustard if desired and serve.

Nutrition: Calories: 308 - Fat: 20.8g - Carbs: 3g - Protein: 26g.

133. Turkey Breast with Fennel and Celery

Preparation Time: 10 minutes
Cooking Time: 15 minutes
Servings: 3
Ingredients:

- 2lb. boneless and skinless turkey breast
- 1 cup fennel bulb, chopped
- 1 cup celery with leaves, chopped
- ¼ cup chicken stock
- ¼ tsp pepper
- ¼ tsp garlic powder

Directions:

1. Throw all ingredients in your pressure cooker. Give it a good stir and seal the lid. Cook for 14 minutes at High. Do a quick pressure release. Shred the turkey with two forks.

Nutrition: Calories: 272 - Carbs: 7g - Fat: 4g - Protein: 48g.

134.   Tangy Chicken with Scallions

Preparation Time: 10 minutes
Cooking Time: 40 minutes
Servings: 4
Ingredients:
- Butter, melted
- 1lb. chicken thighs
- White wine
- 1 garlic clove, sliced
- 1 tablespoon fresh scallions, chopped

Directions:
1. Arrange the chicken drumettes on a foil-lined baking pan. Brush with melted butter.
2. Add in the garlic and wine. Spice with salt and black pepper to taste. Bake in the preheated oven at 400°F for about 30 minutes or until internal temperature reaches about 165°F.
3. Serve garnished with scallions and enjoy!

Nutrition: Calories: 209 - Fat: 12.2g - Carbs: 0.4g Protein: 23.2g - Fibre: 1.9g.

135.   Country-Style Chicken Stew

Preparation Time: 20 minutes
Cooking Time: 1 hour
Servings: 6
Ingredients:
- 1lb. chicken thighs
- Butter, room temperature
- 1/2-pound carrots, chopped
- 1 bell pepper, chopped
- 1 Chile pepper, deveined and minced
- 1 cup tomato puree
- Kosher salt and ground black pepper, to taste
- 1/2 teaspoon smoked paprika
- 1 onion, finely chopped
- 1 teaspoon garlic, sliced
- 2 cups vegetable broth
- 1 teaspoon dried basil
- 1 celery, chopped

Directions:
1. Melt the butter in a stockpot over medium-high flame. Sweat the onion and garlic until just tender and fragrant.
2. Reduce the heat to medium-low. Stir in the broth, chicken thighs, and basil; bring to a rolling boil.
3. Add in the remaining Ingredients. Partially cover and let it simmer for 45 to 50 minutes. Shred the meat, discarding the bones; add the chicken back to the pot. Warm through for a minute or so before serving.

Nutrition: Calories: 280 - Fat: 15g - Carbs: 2.5g - Protein: 27g - Fibre: 2.5g.

136.   Chicken Drumsticks with Broccoli and Cheese

Preparation Time: 40 minutes
Cooking Time: 1 hour 15 minutes
Servings: 4
Ingredients:
- 1lb. chicken drumsticks
- 1lb. broccoli, broken into florets
- 2 cups cheddar cheese, shredded
- 1/2 teaspoon dried oregano
- 1/2 teaspoon dried basil
- Olive oil
- 1 celery, sliced
- 1 cup green onions, chopped
- 1 teaspoon minced green garlic

Directions:
1. Roast the chicken drumsticks in the preheated oven at 380°F for 30 to 35 minutes. Add in the broccoli, celery, green onions, and green garlic.
2. Add in the oregano, basil and olive oil; roast an additional 15 minutes.

Nutrition: Calories: 533 - Fat: 40g - Carbs: 5.4g - Protein: 35g - Fibre: 3.5g.

137.   Greek-Style Saucy Chicken Drumettes

Preparation Time: 25 minutes
Cooking Time: 50 minutes
Servings: 6
Ingredients:

- 1 ½ pounds chicken drumettes
- 1/2 cup port wine
- 1/2 cup onions, chopped
- Garlic cloves, minced
- 1 teaspoon tzatziki spice mix
- 1 cup double cream
- Butter
- Sea salt and crushed mixed peppercorns, to season

Directions:

1. Melt the butter in an oven-proof skillet over a moderate heat; then, cook the chicken for about 8 minutes.
2. Add in the onions, garlic, wine, tzatziki spice mix, double cream, salt, and pepper.
3. Bake in the preheated oven at 375°F for 35 to 40 minutes (a meat thermometer should register 165°F).

Nutrition: Calories: 333 - Fat: 20g - Carbs: 2g - Protein: 33.5g - Fibre: 0.2g.

138.   Autumn Chicken Soup with Root Vegetables

Preparation Time: 10 minutes
Cooking Time: 25 minutes
Servings: 4
Ingredients:

- 2 cups chicken broth
- 1 cup full-fat milk
- 1 cup double cream
- 1/2 cup turnip, chopped
- 1lb. chicken drumsticks, boneless and cut into small pieces
- Salt and pepper, to taste
- 1 tablespoon butter
- 1 teaspoon garlic, finely minced
- 1 carrot, chopped
- 1/2 parsnip, chopped
- 1/2 celery
- 1 whole egg

Directions:

1. Melt the butter in a heavy-bottomed pot over medium-high heat; sauté the garlic until aromatic or about 1 minute. Add in the vegetables and continue to cook until they've softened.
2. Add in the chicken and cook until it is no longer pink for about 4 minutes. Season with salt and pepper.
3. Pour in the chicken broth, milk, and heavy cream and bring it to a boil.
4. Reduce the heat. Partially cover and continue to simmer for 20 to 25 minutes longer. Afterwards, fold the beaten egg and stir until it is well incorporated.

Nutrition: Calories: 342 - Fat: 22.4g - Carbs: 6.3g Protein: 25g - Fibre: 1.3g.

139.   Herbed Chicken Breasts

Preparation Time: 10 minutes
Cooking Time: 40 minutes
Servings: 8
Ingredients:

- 2lb. chicken breasts
- 1 italian pepper, deveined and thinly sliced
- Black olives, pitted
- 1 ½ cups vegetable broth
- Garlic cloves, pressed
- Olive oil
- 1 tablespoon Old Sub Sailor
- Salt, to taste

Directions:

1. Rub the chicken with the garlic and Old Sub Sailor; salt to taste. Heat the oil in a frying pan over a moderately high heat.
2. Sear the chicken until it is browned on all sides, about 5 minutes.
3. Add in the pepper, olives, and vegetable broth and bring it to boil. Reduce the heat simmer and continue to cook, partially covered, for 30 to 35 minutes.

Nutrition: Calories: 306 - Fat: 17.8g - Carbs: 1g - Protein: 32g - Fibre: 0.2g.

140. Chicken burger with bluefin cheese

Preparation Time: 30 minutes
Cooking Time: 15 minutes
Servings: 4
Ingredients:

- 14oz. free range chicken fillet
- Argentinian grill spices
- 1.8oz. Bleu d'Auvergne
- 1.8oz cream cheese natural
- 4 sandwiches
- 10oz. grilled red peppers in a pot
- 14oz. rivolo cherry tomatoes
- 0.7oz. fresh parsley
- 1 jalapeño pepper
- 1 baby romole lettuce

Equipment

- food processor
- 1 grill pan

Directions:

1. Put the free-range chicken fillet, herbs and salt in the food processor and grind almost fine.
2. Form the citizens with moist hands. Heat the grill pan and grill the burgers in approx. 12 minutes. Turn halfway.
3. Crumble the cheese and mix with the cream cheese. Divide this cheese mixture over the burgers for the last 3 minutes and let it melt.
4. Drain the grilled red pepper, but collect 2 tbsp oil (for 4 people). Cut the pepper into strips.
5. Cut the cherry tomatoes in quarters and the parsley fine.
6. Mix the rest of the Argentinian grill spices with the collected oil, pepper and salt.
7. Mix the pepper strips, cherry tomatoes, parsley and herb oil in a bowl.
8. Cut the stalk of the jalapeño pepper, remove the seeds and cut the flesh into thin rings.
9. Cut the buns open. Remove the leaves from the baby cream salad and spread over the bottom halves of the buns.
10. Place the chicken burger, the cheese mixture and the pepper rings in

succession. Put the top of the buns on top and serve together with the salad.

Nutrition: Calories: 465 - Fat: 6g - Carbs: 41g - Protein: 35g - Fibre: 6g.

141. Creamy Mustard Chicken with Shirataki

Preparation Time: 20 minutes
Cooking Time: 30 minutes
Servings: 4
Ingredients:

- 8oz. packs angel hair shirataki
- 1lb. chicken breasts, cut into strips
- 1 cup chopped mustard greens
- 1 yellow bell pepper, sliced
- 1 tbsp olive oil
- 1 yellow onion, finely sliced
- 1 garlic clove, minced
- 1 tbsp wholegrain mustard
- 1 tbsp heavy cream
- 1 tbsp chopped parsley

Directions:

1. Boil 2 cups of water in a medium pot.
2. Strain the shirataki pasta and rinse well under hot running water. Allow proper draining and pour the shirataki pasta into the boiling water.
3. Cook for 3 minutes and strain again. Place a dry skillet and stir-fry the shirataki pasta until visibly dry, 1-2 minutes; set aside.
4. Heat olive oil in a skillet, season the chicken with salt and pepper and cook for 8-10 minutes; set aside. Stir in onion, bell pepper, and garlic and cook until softened, 5 minutes.
5. Mix in mustard and heavy cream; simmer for 2 minutes and mix in the chicken and mustard greens for 2 minutes. Stir in shirataki pasta, garnish with parsley and serve.

Nutrition: Calories: 692 - Carbs: 15g - Fat: 38g - Protein: 65g.

142. Duck and Eggplant Casserole

Preparation Time: 10 minutes
Cooking Time: 45 minutes
Servings: 4
Ingredients:

- 1lb. ground duck meat
- 1 ½ tablespoons ghee, melted
- 1/3 cup double cream
- ½ lb. eggplant, peeled and sliced
- 1 ½ cups almond flour
- Salt and black pepper, to taste
- 1/2 teaspoon fennel seeds
- 1/2 teaspoon oregano, dried
- 3 eggs

Directions:

1. Mix the almond flour with salt, black, fennel seeds, and oregano. Fold in one egg and the melted ghee and whisk to combine well.
2. Press the crust into the bottom of a lightly oiled pie pan. Cook the ground duck until no longer pink for about 3 minutes, stirring continuously.
3. Whisk the remaining eggs and double cream. Fold in the browned meat and stir until everything is well incorporated. Pour the mixture into the prepared crust. Top with the eggplant slices.
4. Bake for about 40 minutes. Cut into four pieces.

Nutrition: Calories: 562 - Fat: 49.5g - Carbs: 6.7g Protein: 22.5g - Fibre: 2g.

143. Old-Fashioned Turkey Chowder

Preparation Time: 15 minutes
Cooking Time: 35 minutes
Servings: 4
Ingredients:

- Olive oil
- 2 tablespoons yellow onions, chopped
- Cloves garlic, roughly chopped
- ½ lb. leftover roast turkey, shredded and skin removed
- 1 teaspoon mediterranean spice mix
- 2 cups chicken bone broth
- 1 ½ cups milk

- 1/2 cup double cream
- 1 egg, lightly beaten
- 2 tablespoons dry sherry

Directions:

1. Heat the olive oil in a heavy-bottomed pot over a moderate flame. Sauté the onion and garlic until they've softened.
2. Stir in the leftover roast turkey, Mediterranean spice mix, and chicken bone broth; bring to a rapid boil. Partially cover and continue to cook for 20 to 25 minutes.
3. Turn the heat to simmer. Pour in the milk and double cream and continue to cook until it has reduced slightly.
4. Fold in the egg and dry sherry; continue to simmer, stirring frequently, for a further 2 minutes.

Nutrition: Calories: 350 - Fat: 25.8g - Carbs: 5.5g Protein: 20g - Fibre: 0.1g.

144. Cheese and Prosciutto Chicken Roulade

Preparation Time: 15 minutes
Cooking Time: 35 minutes
Servings: 2
Ingredients:

- 1/2 cup Ricotta cheese
- 4 slices of prosciutto
- 1lb. chicken fillet
- 1 tablespoon fresh coriander, chopped
- Salt and ground black pepper, to taste pepper
- 1 teaspoon cayenne pepper

Directions:

1. Season the chicken fillet with salt and pepper. Spread the Ricotta cheese over the chicken fillet; sprinkle with the fresh coriander.
2. Roll up and cut into 4 pieces. Wrap each piece with one slice of prosciutto; secure with a kitchen twine.
3. Place the wrapped chicken in a parchment-lined baking pan. Now, bake in the preheated oven at 385°F for about 30 minutes.

Nutrition: Calories: 499 - Fat: 18.9g - Fat: 5.7g - Protein: 41.6g - Fibre: 0.6g.

145.   Chicken with Avocado Sauce

Preparation Time: 10 minutes
Cooking Time: 20 minutes
Servings: 4
Ingredients:
- 1lb. chicken wings, boneless, cut into bite-size chunks
- Olive oil
- Sea salt and pepper, to your liking
- 2 eggs
- 1 teaspoon onion powder
- 1 teaspoon hot paprika
- 1/3 teaspoon mustard seeds
- 1/3 cup almond meal

For the Sauce:
- 1/2 cup mayonnaise
- 1/2 medium avocado
- 1/2 teaspoon sea salt
- 1 teaspoon green garlic, minced

Directions:
1. Pat dry the chicken wings with a paper towel.
2. Thoroughly combine the almond meal, salt, pepper, onion powder, paprika, and mustard seeds.
3. Whisk the eggs in a separate dish. Dredge the chicken chunks into the whisked eggs, then in the almond meal mixture.
4. In a frying pan, heat the oil over a moderate heat; once hot, fry the chicken for about 10 minutes, stirring continuously to ensure even cooking.
5. Make the sauce by whisking all of the sauce Ingredients.

Nutrition: Calories: 370 - Fat: 25g - Carbs: 4g - Protein: 31.4g - Fibre: 2.6g.

146.   Chinese Bok Choy and Turkey Soup

Preparation Time: 15 minutes
Cooking Time: 40 minutes
Servings: 8
Ingredients:
- 1/2lb. baby Bok choy, sliced into quarters lengthwise
- 1lb. pounds turkey carcass
- 1 tablespoon olive oil
- 1/2 cup leeks, chopped
- 1 celery rib, chopped
- 4 carrots, sliced
- 3 cups turkey stock
- Himalayan salt and black pepper, to taste

Directions:
1. In a heavy-bottomed pot, heat the olive oil until sizzling. Once hot, sauté the celery, carrots, leek and Bok choy for about 6 minutes.
2. Add the salt, pepper, turkey, and stock; bring to a boil.
3. Turn the heat to simmer. Continue to cook, partially covered, for about 35 minutes.

Nutrition: Calories: 211 - Fat: 12g - Carbs: 3g - Protein: 24g - Fibre: 0.9g.

147.   Lovely Pulled Chicken Egg Bites

Preparation Time: 15 minutes
Cooking Time: 30 minutes
Servings: 4
Ingredients:
- 1 tbsp butter
- 1 chicken breast
- 1 tbsp chopped green onions
- ½ tsp red chilli flakes
- Eggs dipende quandi buchi ci sono
- ¼ cup grated Monterey Jack

Directions:
1. Preheat oven to 400°F. Line a 12-hole muffin tin with cupcake liners. Melt butter in a skillet over medium heat and cook the chicken until brown on each side, 10 minutes.
2. Transfer to a plate and shred with 2 forks. Divide between muffin holes along with green onions and red chilli flakes.
3. Crack an egg into each muffin hole and scatter the cheese on top. Bake for 15 minutes until eggs set. Serve.

Nutrition: Calories: 393 - Carbs 0.5g - Fat 27g - Protein 34g.

148. Festive Turkey Rouladen

Preparation Time: 15 minutes
Cooking Time: 30 minutes
Servings: 5
Ingredients:

- 2lb.turkey fillet, marinated and cut into 10 pieces
- Strips prosciutto
- 1/2 teaspoon chilli powder
- 1 teaspoon marjoram
- 1 sprig rosemary, finely chopped
- Dry white wine
- 1 teaspoon garlic, finely minced
- 1 ½ tablespoons butter, room temperature
- 1 tablespoon Dijon mustard
- Sea salt and freshly ground black pepper, to your liking

Directions:

1. Start by preheating your oven to 430°F.
2. Pat the turkey dry and cook in hot butter for about 3 minutes per side. Add in the mustard, chilli powder, marjoram, rosemary, wine, and garlic.
3. Continue to cook for 2 minutes more. Wrap each turkey piece into one prosciutto strip and secure with toothpicks.
4. Roast in the preheated oven for about 30 minutes.

Nutrition: Calories: 286 - Fat: 9.7g - Carbs: 7g - Protein: 40g - Fibre: 0.3g.

149. Herby Chicken Meatloaf

Preparation Time: 20 minutes
Cooking Time: 30 minutes
Servings: 6
Ingredients:

- ½ lb. ground chicken
- 1 tbsp flaxseed meal
- 2 large eggs
- Olive oil
- 1 lemon,1 tbsp juiced
- ¼ cup chopped parsley
- ¼ cup chopped oregano
- Garlic cloves, minced
- Lemon slices to garnish

Directions:

1. Preheat oven to 400°F. In a bowl, combine ground chicken and flaxseed meal; set aside. In a small bowl, whisk the eggs with olive oil, lemon juice, parsley, oregano, and garlic.
2. Pour the mixture onto the chicken mixture and mix well. Spoon into a greased loaf pan and press to fit. Bake for 40 minutes.
3. Remove the pan, drain the liquid, and let cool a bit. Slice, garnish with lemon slices, and serve.

Nutrition: Calories: 362 - Carbs: 1.3g - Fat: 24g Protein: 35g.

Chapter 12. Seafood

150. Low Carbs Poached Eggs with Tuna Salad

Preparation time: 10 minutes
Cooking time: 20 minutes
Servings: 4
Ingredients:
Tuna salad:

- 4oz. tuna in olive oil, rinsed and drained
- ⅓ cup chopped celery stalks
- ½ red onion
- ½ cup mayonnaise, intermittent-friendly
- 1 teaspoon Dijon mustard
- Juice and zest of ½ lemon
- Salt and freshly ground black pepper, to taste
- Olive oil
- 2oz. leafy greens or lettuce
- 2oz. cherry tomatoes, chopped

Poached eggs: Spostato

- 4 eggs
- 1 teaspoon salt
- White wine vinegar or white vinegar

Directions:

1. Chop the tuna and mix it in a bowl with the other ingredients for the salad. You can make it ahead of time and keep it in the refrigerator. The flavor will enhance with time.
2. Bring a pot of water to a boil over medium heat. Add the vinegar and salt, then stir the water in circles to create a swirl using a spoon. Crack the eggs into the pot, one at a time.
3. Let simmer for 3 minutes and use a slotted spoon to remove it from the water.
4. Transfer the eggs to the bowl of tuna salad and drizzle with olive oil. Gently toss until everything is combined.
5. Serve them with leafy greens and cherry tomatoes on the side.

Nutrition: Calories: 534 - Fat: 40.5g - Carbs: 7.2g Fibre: 1.4g -Protein: 34g.

151. Blackened Trout

Preparation time: 20 minutes
Cooking time: 10 minutes
Servings: 6
Ingredients:

- 2 teaspoons dry mustard
- 1 tablespoon paprika
- 1 teaspoon ground cumin
- 1 teaspoon cayenne pepper
- 1 teaspoon white pepper
- 1 teaspoon black pepper
- 1 teaspoon dried thyme
- 1 teaspoon salt
- ¾ cup unsalted butter, melted
- 4oz. trout fillets
- 1 tablespoon olive oil

Directions:

1. Combine the dry mustard, paprika, cumin, cayenne pepper, white pepper, black pepper, thyme, and salt in a medium bowl. Stir to combine and set aside.
2. Put ¾ cup butter on a platter, then dredge the trout fillets into the butter to coat evenly. Sprinkle with the spicy mixture, gently pressing the mixture into the fillets.
3. Heat the olive oil in a skillet over medium-high heat, then add the fillets. Cook the fish for about 2 to 3 minutes per side, turning occasionally, or until the fish is lightly browned on the edges.
4. Remove from the heat and serve warm.

Nutrition: Calories: 328 - Fat: 25.0g - Carbs: 1.7g Fibre: 0.8g - Protein: 24g.

152. Trout Fillets with Lemony Yogurt Sauce

Preparation time: 12 minutes
Cooking time: 8 to 10 minutes
Servings: 4
Ingredients:

- 1 cup plain Greek yogurt
- 1 cucumber, shredded
- 1 teaspoon lemon zest
- 1 tablespoon extra-virgin olive oil
- Salt and freshly ground black pepper, to taste
- 2 tablespoons fresh dill weed, chopped
- 1 pinch lemon pepper
- 6oz. rainbow trout fillets

Directions:

1. Mix the yogurt, cucumber, lemon zest, olive oil, salt, and pepper in a bowl. Stir thoroughly and set aside.
2. Preheat the oven to 400°F.
3. Sprinkle the lemon pepper on top and arrange the fillets in a greased baking dish.
4. Bake in the preheated oven for about 8 to 10 minutes or until fork tender.
5. Remove from the oven and serve the fish alongside the yogurt sauce.

Nutrition: Calories: 281 - Fat: 11.4g - Carbs: 5.3g Fibre: 0.7g - Protein: 37.6g.

153. Classic Shrimp Scampi

Preparation time: 30 minutes
Cooking time: 15 minutes
Servings: 4
Ingredients:

- Cloves garlic, minced
- ½ cup butter, melted
- ½ cup dry white wine
- 2lb. medium shrimp, peeled and deveined
- Green onions, chopped

Directions:

1. Preheat the oven to 400°F.
2. In a bowl, combine the garlic, butter, wine, and shrimp. Stir thoroughly.

3. Arrange the shrimp in a greased baking dish. Place the baking dish in the oven and bake for about 8 minutes until the shrimp is opaque.
4. Remove from the oven and serve the shrimp with green onions on top.

Nutrition: Calories: 209 - Fat: 2.2g - Carbs: 1.6g Fibre: 0.2g -Protein: 46g.

154. Snow Crab Clusters with Garlic Butter

Preparation time: 5 minutes
Cooking time: 15 minutes
Servings: 2
Ingredients:

- 1lb. snow crab clusters, thawed if necessary
- ¼ cup butter
- 1 clove garlic, minced
- 1½ teaspoons dried parsley
- ⅛ teaspoon salt
- ¼ teaspoon ground black pepper

Directions:

1. On the cutting board, cut a slit lengthwise into the shell of each crab. Set aside.
2. In a skillet, melt the butter over medium heat. Add the garlic and cook for 2 minutes until tender. Add the parsley, salt, and pepper, then cook for 1 minute more. Stir in the crab and simmer for 5 to 6 minutes.
3. Remove from the heat and serve on a plate.

Nutrition: Calories: 222 - Fat: 4g - Carbs: 0.8g - Fibre: 0.1g - Protein: 45.7g.

155.   Intermittent Taco Fishbowl

Preparation time: 5 minutes
Cooking time: 10 minutes
Servings: 4
Ingredients:
Dressing:
- ½ cup intermittent-friendly mayonnaise
- Lime juice
- 1 teaspoon hot sauce
- ½ teaspoon garlic powder
- Salt and freshly ground black pepper, to taste

Main meal:
- ½lb. green cabbage or red cabbage
- ½ yellow onion
- 1 tomato
- 1 avocado
- Salt and ground black pepper, to taste
- 4 tablespoons olive oil, divided
- 10oz. white fish, patted dry
- 1 tablespoon tex-mex seasoning
- Fresh cilantro, for garnish
- Lime, for garnish

Directions:
1. In a bowl, mix the ingredients for the dressing before frying the fish, so the flavors have time to develop. Allow to sit at room temperature or keep in the refrigerator.
2. With a sharp knife or mandolin, shred or slice all vegetables finely except the avocado. Split the avocado in half and remove the pit. Slice the avocado thinly and using a spoon to scoop avocado slices out of the skin. Season the vegetables and avocado slices with salt and pepper on a plate, then drizzle with 2 tablespoons olive oil. Toss well and set aside.
3. Rub both sides of white fish with salt, pepper, and Tex-Mex seasoning.
4. In a skillet, add the remaining olive oil. Fry the fish in olive oil over medium heat for 3 to 4 minutes on both sides, or until the fish flakes easily with a fork.
5. Transfer the vegetable mixture to a serving bowl. Top with the fish and pour over the dressing. Garnish with fresh cilantro and lime before serving.

Nutrition: Calories: 489 - Fat: 43g - Carbs: 14.2g Fibre: 5.6g - Protein: 15g.

156.   Smoked Salmon and Lettuce Bites

Preparation time: 20 minutes
Cooking time: 0
Servings: 6
Ingredients:
- 7oz. smoked salmon, cut into small pieces
- 8oz. cream cheese
- ⅓ tablespoon mayonnaise, intermittent-friendly
- 2 tablespoons chopped fresh dill or fresh chives
- ½ lemon, zested
- ¼ teaspoon ground black pepper
- 2oz. lettuce, for serving

Directions:
1. Add the cream cheese, mayonnaise, fresh dill, lemon zest, and pepper in a bowl. Stir to combine well.
2. Lay the lettuce on a clean work surface. Top with the salmon pieces and pour the cream cheese mixture over. Serve immediately.

Nutrition: Calories: 179 - Fat: 15g - Carbs: 3.3g - Fibre: 1.1g - Protein: 8.6g.

157. Intermittent Chilli-Covered Salmon with Spinach

Preparation time: 5 minutes
Cooking time: 20 minutes
Servings: 4
Ingredients:

- ¼ cup olive oil
- 1½ pounds salmon, in pieces
- Salt and freshly ground black pepper, to taste
- 1oz. parmesan cheese, grated finely
- 1 tablespoon chilli paste
- ½ cup sour cream
- 1lb. fresh spinach

Directions:

1. Preheat oven to 400°F.
2. Grease the baking dish with half of the olive oil, season the salmon with pepper and salt, and put in the baking dish, skin-side down.
3. Combine Parmesan cheese, chilli paste and sour cream. Then spread them on the salmon fillets.
4. Bake for 20 minutes, or until the salmon flakes easily with a fork or it becomes opaque.
5. Heat the remaining olive oil in a nonstick skillet, sauté the spinach until it's wilted, about a couple of minutes, and season with pepper and salt.
6. Serve with the oven-baked salmon immediately.

Nutrition: Calories: 461 - Fat: 28.5g - Carbs: 8g - Fibre: 2.8g - Protein: 42.6g.

158. Intermittent Egg Butter with Avocado and Smoked Salmon

Preparation time: 5 minutes
Cooking time: 15 minutes
Servings: 4
Ingredients:

- 4 eggs
- ½ teaspoon sea salt
- ¼ teaspoon ground black pepper
- 5oz. butter, at room temperature
- 4oz. smoked salmon
- 1 tablespoon fresh parsley, chopped finely
- Avocados
- Olive oil

Directions:

1. Put the eggs in a pot and cover them with cold water. Then put the pot on the stove without a lid and bring it to a boil.
2. Lower the heat and let it simmer for 6 to 9 minutes. Then remove eggs from the water and put them in a bowl with cold water.
3. Peel the eggs and cut them finely. Use a fork to mix the eggs and butter. Then season to taste with pepper, salt.
4. Serve the egg butter with slices of smoked salmon, finely chopped parsley, and a side of diced avocado tossed in olive oil.

Nutrition: Calories: 638 - Fat: 61g - Carbs: 9.8g - Fibre: 6.8g - Protein: 16.5g.

159.   Intermittent Baked Salmon with Butter and Lemon Slices

Preparation time: 10 minutes
Cooking time: 25 minutes
Servings: 6
Ingredients:
- 1 tablespoon olive oil
- 2lb. salmon
- 1 teaspoon sea salt
- Freshly ground black pepper, to taste
- 7oz. butter
- 1 lemon

Directions:
1. Start by preheating the oven to 400°F.
2. In a large baking dish, spray it with olive oil. Then add the salmon, skin-side down. Season with salt and pepper.
3. Cut the lemon into thin slices and place them on the upper side of the salmon. Cut the butter in thin slices and spread them on top of the lemon slices.
4. Put the dish in the heated oven and bake on the middle rack for about 25 minutes, or until the salmon flakes easily with a fork.
5. Melt the rest of the butter in a small saucepan until it bubbles. Then remove from heat and let cool a little. Consider adding some lemon juice on the melted cool butter.
6. Serve the fish with the lemon butter.

Nutrition: Calories: 474 - Fat: 37.6g - Carbs: 0.7g Fibre: 0.1g - Protein: 32.6g.

160.   Grilled Tuna Salad with Garlic Sauce

Preparation time: 10 minutes
Cooking time: 15 minutes
Servings: 4
Ingredients:
Garlic dressing:
- ⅔ cup intermittent-friendly mayonnaise
- 2 tablespoons water
- 2 teaspoons garlic powder
- Salt and freshly ground black pepper, to taste

Tuna salad:
- 4 eggs
- 8oz. green asparagus
- 1 tablespoon olive oil
- ¾ pound fresh tuna, in slices
- 4oz. leafy greens
- 2oz. cherry tomatoes
- ½ red onion
- Pumpkin seeds
- Salt and freshly ground black pepper, to taste

Directions:
1. Mix the ingredients together for the garlic dressing. And set them aside.
2. Put the eggs in boiling water for 8 to 10 minutes. Cooling in cold water would facilitate the peeling.
3. Slice the asparagus into lengths and rapidly fry them inside a hot pan with no oil or butter. Then set them aside.
4. Rub the tuna with oil and fry or grill for 2 to 3 minutes on each side. Season with salt and pepper.
5. Put the leafy greens, asparagus, peeled eggs cut in halves, tomatoes and thinly sliced onion into a plate.
6. Finally, cut the tuna into slices and spread the slices evenly over the salad. Pour the dressing on top and add some pumpkin seeds.

Nutrition: Calories: 397 - Fat: 27.1g - Carbs: 8.3g Fibre: 2.8g -Protein: 30g.

161. Grilled White Fish with Zucchini and Kale Pesto

Preparation time: 10 minutes
Cooking time: 15 minutes
Servings: 4
Ingredients:
Kale pesto:
- 3oz. kale, chopped
- 1 garlic clove
- Lemon juice
- 2oz. walnuts, shelled
- ½ teaspoon salt
- ¼ teaspoon ground black pepper
- Olive oil

Fish and zucchini:
- 2 zucchinis, rinsed and drained, cut into slices
- Olive oil, divided
- Salt and freshly ground black pepper, to taste
- 1 teaspoon lemon juice
- 1½ pounds white fish (such as cod), thawed at room temperature, if frozen

Directions:
1. Make the kale pesto: Add the kale to the food processor with the garlic, lemon juice, and walnuts and blend, then sprinkle with salt and pepper for seasoning, and then add the olive oil and blend until the mixture becomes creamy and set aside until ready to serve.
2. Rub the zucchini slices with 1 tablespoon of olive oil, salt, pepper, and lemon juice and set aside.
3. Grease a nonstick skillet with remaining olive oil, and heat over medium-high heat.
4. Grill the fish in the skillet for 3 minutes on each side. Sprinkle with salt and black pepper, and serve with zucchini and kale pesto immediately.

Nutrition: Calories: 321 - Fat: 19.5g - Carbs: 8.1g Fibre: 2.8g - Protein: 30.3g.

162. Coconut Intermittent Salmon and Napa Cabbage

Preparation time: 10 minutes
Cooking time: 20 minutes
Servings: 4
Ingredients:
- 1¼ pounds salmon
- 1 tablespoon coconut oil
- 1 teaspoon sea salt
- ½ teaspoon onion powder
- 1 teaspoon turmeric
- 2oz. unsweetened shredded coconut
- Olive oil, for frying
- 1¼ pounds napa cabbage
- Salt and freshly ground black pepper, to taste
- 4oz. butter
- Lemon, for serving

Directions:
1. On a wooden board, cut the salmon into 1×1-inch pieces. Then rub coconut oil on salmon pieces. Place the pieces in a medium bowl and set aside.
2. Prepare a mixture of salt, onion powder, turmeric, and unsweetened shredded coconut, finely mix the mixture. Meanwhile, put the salmon pieces into this creamy mixture to get a good coating.
3. In a nonstick frying pan with 4 tablespoons of olive oil on medium heat. Fry the seasoned salmon pieces with coconut mixture for about 4 to 7 minutes in a pan, stirring every 2 minutes. Leave it in the pan until golden brown, or until soft.
4. Meanwhile, prepare and cut the cabbage into wedges. Fry the cabbage in a saucepan with butter until it turns into a light creamy liquid. On a platter, pour the cabbage liquid and generously season with salt and pepper.
5. In a dish decorated with lemon slices, place the fried salmon and pour the creamy cabbage liquid and top with wedges of lemon. Serve warm!

Nutrition: Calories: 628 - Fat: 52.9g - Carbs: 7.1g Fibre: 1.6g - Protein: 32.7g.

163. Crispy Intermittent Creamy Fish Casserole

Preparation time: 25 minutes
Cooking time: 30 minutes
Servings: 4
Ingredients:

- 1 head broccoli, cut into florets
- Olive oil
- 1 teaspoon salt
- ¼ teaspoon freshly ground black pepper
- 2 scallions, chopped
- 1oz. melted butter, for greasing the casserole dish
- 1 tablespoon parsley, finely chopped
- 1¼ cups heavy whipping cream
- 1 tablespoon Dijon mustard
- 1½ pounds white fish, in serving- pieces
- 3oz. butter slices, under room temperature

Directions:

1. Preheat the oven to 400°F.
2. Heat the olive oil in a nonstick skillet over medium heat.
3. Add the broccoli to the skillet and sauté for 5 to 7 minutes or until tender, then season the broccoli with salt and ground black pepper, add the finely chopped scallions, and sauté for 1 to 2 minutes more.
4. Prepare a casserole dish and grease it with butter to add a tasty level of flavors to the meal. Then pour the sautéed broccoli and scallions in the casserole dish, stir them well until they have a delicious butter smell.
5. In a bowl, mix finely chopped parsley with cream and Dijon mustard and pour the mixture over the casserole dish. Stir until fully incorporated. Then nestle the white fish in the casserole dish. Top them with the butter slices.
6. Cook in the preheated oven for 20 to 30 minutes, or until the fish exudes tender and takes in the flavor from the delicious butter.
7. Remove the casserole dish from the oven and serve the fish and vegetables warm.

Nutrition: Calories: 611 - Fat: 48.3g - Carbs: 13.2g - Fibre: 4.8g - Protein: 34.4g.

164. Creamy Salmon Sauce Zoodles

Preparation time: 15 minutes
Cooking time: 15 minutes
Servings: 4
Ingredients:

- 2lb. zucchini
- Salt and freshly ground black pepper, to taste
- 4oz. cream cheese
- 1 cup heavy whipping cream
- ¼ cup chopped fresh basil
- 1lb. smoked salmon
- 1 lime, juiced
- Olive oil

Directions:

1. Cut the zucchini after washing it thoroughly into thin slices with a sharp knife.
2. Prepare a colander to filter the zucchini, add a little salt and toss to coat well. Leave them sit for 7 to 12 minutes. Gently press the mixture to get rid of excess salted water.
3. Meanwhile, mix the cream cheese with lemon juice, chopped fresh basil in a bowl. Set aside until ready to serve.
4. Cut the salmon into thin slices and sprinkle with salt and pepper. Add the salmon to an oiled skillet and fry over medium-high heat for 8 minutes or until the salmon is opaque and tender on both sides. Then add zucchini spirals and cook for 2 minutes until soft.
5. Serve the recipe on a large plate with the cream sauce.

Nutrition: Calories: 444 - Fat: 33.4g - Carbs: 10g Fibre: 2.6g - Protein: 29.3g.

165. Cheesy Verde Shrimp

Preparation time: 10 minutes
Cooking time: 10 minutes
Servings: 4
Ingredients:

- Olive oil
- Garlic cloves, minced
- ¼ cup scallions, chopped
- 1lb. fresh shrimps, deveined, and peeled
- ½ cup parsley, chopped
- ½ cup Parmesan cheese, grated

Directions:

1. In a large skillet, heat the olive oil over medium heat.
2. Add the garlic and chopped scallions and sauté briefly, making sure the garlic does not turn brown.
3. Add the shrimps and cook until they become opaque. Sprinkle chopped parsley over the shrimp.
4. Remove cooked shrimps from heat. Serve on a dish and sprinkle with grated cheese.

Nutrition: Calories: 215 - Fat: 10.9g - Carbs: 3.2g Fibre: 0.4g - Protein: 26.8g.

166. Best Marinated Grilled Shrimp

Preparation time: 15 minutes
Cooking time: 6 minutes
Servings: 4
Ingredients:

- ⅓ cup olive oil
- Cloves garlic, minced
- Chopped fresh basil
- Red wine vinegar
- ½ teaspoon salt
- ¼ teaspoon cayenne pepper
- 2lb. fresh shrimp, peeled and deveined
- 1 tablespoon olive oil, for greasing
- Wooden skewers, soaked for at least 25-30 minutes

Directions:

1. Mix the olive oil, garlic, basil, red wine vinegar, salt, and cayenne in a large bowl. Stir in the shrimp and toss to coat well.
2. Cover the bowl with plastic wrap, then place in the refrigerator to marinate for 1 hour.
3. Preheat the grill to medium heat and lightly spray the grill grates with olive oil spray.
4. Thread the shrimp onto skewers, piercing once near the tail and once near the head, discarding the marinade.
5. Grill for 6 minutes, flipping occasionally, or until the shrimp is opaque.
6. Allow to cool for about 3 minutes and serve hot.

Nutrition: Calories: 278 - Fat: 14.6g - Carbs: 0.9g Fibre: 0.1g - Protein: 36.4g.

167. Salmon Fillets Baked with Dijon

Preparation time: 10 minutes
Cooking time: 15 minutes
Servings: 4
Ingredients:

- 4oz. salmon fillets
- ¼ cup butter, melted
- Dijon mustard
- Salt and freshly ground black pepper, to taste
- ⅛ cup coconut flour

Directions:

1. Preheat the oven to 375°F and line a baking pan with aluminum foil.
2. In a bowl, mix the salmon fillets, butter, mustard, salt and pepper. Stir well until the salmon is fully coated.
3. Place the salmon in the baking pan, then evenly sprinkle the coconut flour on top.
4. Transfer the pan into the preheated oven and bake until the salmon easily flakes when tested with a fork, about 15 minutes.
5. Remove from the oven and cool for 4-5 minutes before serving.

Nutrition: Calories: 484 - Fat: 21.6g - Carbs: 2.7g Fibre: 0.5g - Protein: 70.1g.

168. Salmon With Garlic Dijon Mustard

Preparation time: 15 minutes
Cooking time: 20 minutes
Servings: 4
Ingredients:
- 1 tablespoon olive oil
- ⅓ cup Dijon mustard
- 6oz. salmon fillets
- 1 red onion, thinly sliced
- Large cloves garlic, thinly sliced
- Salt and freshly ground black pepper, to taste
- 1 teaspoon dried tarragon

Directions:
1. Preheat the oven to 400°F and grease a baking pan with olive oil.
2. Generously rub the Dijon mustard all over the salmon, then place the salmon in the pan, skin-side down.
3. Put the onion slices and garlic cloves on the salmon fillets. Sprinkle with salt, pepper, and tarragon.
4. Arrange the pan in the preheated oven and bake for 20 minutes, or until the salmon easily flakes when tested with a fork.
5. Remove from the heat and serve on a plate.

Nutrition: Calories: 265 - Fat: 11.6g - Carbs: 2.8g Fibre: 1.1g - Protein: 36g.

169. Delicious Intermittent Ceviche

Preparation time: 15 minutes
Cooking time: 0 minutes
Servings: 4
Ingredients:
- 1lb. skinless white fish, cut into ½-inch cubes
- ½ red onion, thinly sliced
- 1 fresh jalapeño, deseeded and thinly sliced
- ¼ red bell pepper, thinly sliced
- 1 tablespoon salt
- ¾ cup lime juice, plus more as needed

For serving:
- Lime juice
- 1 lime, cut into wedges

- Olive oil
- Fresh cilantro, minced

Directions:
1. Prepare a dish with a lid to put the skinless white fish, then add the onions, jalapeño, thinly sliced bell pepper, and salt. Toss to coat the fish well. Pour the lime juice over.
2. Leave the fish in the fridge for about 3 hours for infusing.
3. Take the fish and vegetables out of the fridge and discard the marinade. Rinse the fish and vegetables thoroughly with cold water.
4. Place the fish on a serving dish, then drizzle with olive oil and lemon juice. Spread the fresh cilantro for topping. Serve cold with lime.

Nutrition: Calories: 174 - Fat:7.6g - Carbs: 6.3g - Fibre: 0.6g - Protein: 20.7g.

170. Baked Salmon with Orange Juice

Preparation time: 10 minutes
Cooking time: 10 minutes
Servings: 2
Ingredients:
- ½lb. salmon steak
- 1 orange juice
- Pinch of ginger powder
- Black pepper, to taste
- Salt, to taste
- ½ lemon juice
- 1oz. coconut milk

Directions:
1. Rub salmon steak with spices and let it sit for 15-20 minutes.
2. Take a bowl and squeeze an orange.
3. Squeeze lemon juice as well and mix.
4. Pour milk into the mixture and stir.
5. Take a baking dish and line with aluminum foil.
6. Place teak on it and pour the sauce over steak.
7. Cover with another sheet and bake for 10 minutes at 360°F.
8. Serve and enjoy!

Nutrition: Calories: 300 - Fat: 3g -Carbs: 1g - Protein: 7g - Fibre: 1g.

171. Salmon Croquettes

Preparation Time: 8 minutes
Cooking Time: 7 minutes
Servings: 4
Ingredients:
- 1lb. can red salmon, drained and mashed
- ⅓ cup olive oil
- 2 eggs, beaten
- 1 cup intermittent-friendly breadcrumbs
- ½ bunch parsley, chopped

Directions:
1. Preheat the Air Fryer to 400°F.
2. In a mixing bowl, combine the drained salmon, eggs, and parsley.
3. In a shallow dish, stir together the breadcrumbs and oil to combine well.
4. Mold equal-sized amounts of the mixture into small balls and coat each one with breadcrumbs.
5. Put the croquettes in the fryer's basket and air fry for 6-7 minutes.

Nutrition: Calories: 442 - Protein: 30.5g - Fat: 32.6g - Carbs: 5.3g.

172. Intermittent Salmon in Foil Packets with Pesto

Preparation time: 10 minutes
Cooking time: 20 minutes
Servings: 4
Ingredients:
- 20 tomatoes
- 1lb. salmon fillet
- ½ tsp kosher salt
- ½ cup dry white wine
- 2 tbsp olive oil
- ⅛ tsp ground black pepper
- ¼ cup basil pesto
- Cauliflower rice (optional)

Directions:
1. Put the salmon on a very large tin foil.
2. Sprinkle some salt and pepper.
3. Drizzle a bit of olive oil
4. Arrange the cherry tomatoes around the fish then fold up the foil in such a way that it resembles a mini volcano.
5. Drizzle the white wine over the salmon through the tiny hole at the top.
6. Now seal the top of your volcano and cook on a grill at about 400°F for 10 minutes.
7. Take it out of the grill but leave it sealed for 5 minutes.
8. Open it and glaze the salmon with pesto.
9. Serve with cauliflower rice if you like.

Nutrition Calories: 393 - Fat: 29g - Carbs: 4g - Protein: 27g - Fibre :1g.

173. Low Carbs Soft Shell Crab

Preparation time: 8 minutes
Cooking time: 8 minutes
Servings: 2
Ingredients:
- 2 eggs
- 8 soft shell crabs
- 8oz. of parmesan cheese
- 4 tbsp carolina BBQ sauce

Directions:
1 Shred your parmesan until it's smooth then set it aside.
1. Beat your eggs and set aside.
2. Heat a large pan with half cup of lard to medium heat. Dry the crab with a paper towel.
3. Pour the parmesan into a shallow dish.
4. Pour your eggs into another shallow dish.
5. Dip each crab in the egg dish very lightly then dip the egg coated crab into the Parmesan dish and coat heavily.
6. Fry the crabs in hot oil for about 2 minutes. Flip occasionally until the whole crab is thoroughly cooked.
7. Serve fresh with Carolina BBQ sauce

Nutrition Calories: 388 - Fat: 14g - Protein: 16g Carbs: 2g - Fibre: 1g.

174. Coconut Crab Patties

Preparation time: 3 minutes
Cooking time: 15 minutes
Servings: 2
Ingredients:

- 1 tbsp coconut oil
- 1 tbsp lemon juice
- 1 cup lump crab meat
- 1 tsp Dijon mustard
- 1 egg, beaten
- 1 ½ tbsp coconut flour

Directions:

1. In a bowl to the crabmeat, add all the ingredients, except for the oil; mix well to combine. Make patties out of the mixture.
2. Melt the coconut oil in a skillet over medium heat. Add the crab patties and cook for about 2-3 minutes per side.

Nutrition: Calories: 215 - Fat: 11.5g - Carbs: 3.6g Protein: 15.3g.

175. Low Carbs Oyster Recipe

Preparation time: 10 minutes
Cooking time: 2 minutes
Servings: 2
Ingredients:

- 1 tbsp olive oil
- 12 shucked oysters
- Fresh basil leaves
- 1 tbsp huy fong's garlic chilli paste
- Salt

Directions:

1. Get a small bowl to mix the garlic paste, salt and olive oil.
2. When it's mixed, add the oysters and toss to coat it with the sauce.
3. Spread the basil leaves on a dish. That's going to be your oyster bed.
4. Spread the coated oysters on the basil bed and place the dish on the top rack in then.
5. Turn on the broiler and leave for 3 minutes.
6. Serve hot.

Nutrition: Calories: 204 - Fat: 16g - Carbs: 4g - Protein: 8g.

176. Cheese and Seafood Stuffed Mushrooms

Preparation time: 10 minutes
Cooking time: 55 minutes
Servings: 30
Ingredients:

- ¼ cup paleo mayo
- 1cup chopped cooked shrimp
- ¾ package cream cheese
- 1 can drained crab meat
- ¼ cup parmesan cheese, grated
- ½ teaspoon onion powder
- 1 teaspoon dijon mustard
- ¼ teaspoon garlic powder
- ½ cup sharp cheddar cheese, grated
- 1 tablespoon chopped parsley
- 36 clean large white button mushrooms
- Frank's red hot (This is optional)

Directions:

1. Using parchment paper, line a fairly sized baking sheet
2. Mix all the ingredients except the mushrooms in a mixing bowl and stir gently.
3. Hold the mushrooms in one hand and use a spoon in the other hand to fill the mushroom holes with the mixed ingredients. Put just enough filling to create a tiny mountain on your mushroom.
4. Arrange the stuffed mushrooms on the lined baking sheet and put the sheet in the fridge for about 30 minutes.
5. While that's going on, prep your oven to 375°F.
6. After 30 minutes, transfer the baking sheet to the oven and leave until it looks brownish. This should take about 20 minutes.
7. Remove them from the oven and let them cool for 5 minutes before sprinkling with parsley. Serve.

Nutrition: Calories: 98 - Fat: 6g - Carbs: 2.8g - Protein: 8g.

177. Parmesan Crusted Salmon

Preparation time: 10 minutes
Cooking time: 15 minutes
Servings: 2
Ingredients:

- 1 ½ garlic cloves, minced
- 1lb. salmon fillet
- Salt and black pepper to taste
- ¼ cup parmesan, grated
- 1/8 cup parsley, chopped

Directions:

1. Place the salmon on a lined baking sheet. Season with salt, and pepper. Cover with parchment paper.
2. Place in the oven at 425°F and bake for 10 minutes.
3. Remove the fish and sprinkle with parmesan, parsley, and garlic.
4. Bake again for 5 minutes.
5. Serve.

Nutrition: Calories: 240 - Fat: 12g - Carbs: 0.6g - Protein: 25g.

178. Salmon with Lime Butter Sauce

Preparation Time: 20 minutes
Cooking Time: 10 minutes.
Servings: 2
Ingredients

- 2 salmon fillets
- 1 lime, juiced, divided
- ½ tbsp. minced garlic
- Butter, unsalted
- 1 tbsp. avocado oil

Seasoning:

- 1/4 tsp salt
- 1/4 tsp ground black pepper

Directions:

1. Prepare the fillets and for this, season fillets with salt and black pepper, place them on a shallow dish, drizzle with half of the lime juice and then marinate for 15 minutes.
2. Meanwhile, prepare the lime butter sauce and for this, take a small saucepan place it over medium-low heat, add utter, garlic, and half of the lime juice, stir until mixed, and then bring it to a low boil, set aside until required.
3. Then take a medium skillet pan, place it over medium-high heat, add oil and when hot, place marinated salmon in it, cook for 3 minutes per side and then transfer to a plate.
4. Top each salmon with prepared lime butter sauce and then serve.

Nutrition: Calories: 192 - Fat: 18g - Protein: 6g - Carbs: 4g - Fibre: 0g.

179. Cheesy Baked Mahi-Mahi

Preparation Time: 10 minutes
Cooking Time: 25 minutes.
Servings: 2
Ingredients

- 2 fillets of mahi-mahi
- ½ tsp minced garlic
- 1 tbsp. mayonnaise
- 1 tbsp. grated parmesan cheese
- 1 tbsp. grated mozzarella cheese

Seasoning:

- ½ tsp salt
- ¼ tsp ground black pepper
- 1 tbsp. mustard paste
- ¼ of lime, juiced

Directions:

1. Turn on the oven, then set it to 400°F and let it preheat.
2. Meanwhile, take a baking sheet, line it with foil, place fillets on it and then season with salt and black pepper.
3. Take a small bowl, add mayonnaise, stir in garlic, lime juice and mustard until well mixed and then spread this mixture evenly on fillets.
4. Stir together parmesan cheese and mozzarella cheese, sprinkle it over fillets and then bake for 15 to 20 minutes until thoroughly cooked.
5. Then Turn on the broiler and continue cooking the fillets for 2 to 3 minutes until the top is nicely golden brown.
6. Serve.

Nutrition: Calories: 241 - Fat: 13.6g - Protein: 25g - Carbs: 1.1g - Fibre: 0g.

180.   Shrimp in Curry Sauce

Preparation time: 3 minutes
Cooking time: 15 minutes
Servings: 2
Ingredients:
- ½ ounce grated Parmesan cheese
- 1 egg, beaten
- ¼ tsp curry powder
- 1 tsp almond flour
- 1lb. shrimp, shelled
- 1 tbsp coconut oil

Sauce:
- 1 tbsp curry leaves
- 1 tbsp butter
- ½ onion, diced
- ½ cup heavy cream
- ½ ounce cheddar cheese, shredded

Directions:
1. Combine all dry ingredients for the batter. Melt the coconut oil in a skillet over medium heat. Dip the shrimp in the egg first, and then coat with the dry mixture. Fry until golden and crispy.
2. In another skillet, melt butter. Add onion and cook for 3 minutes. Add curry leaves and cook for 30 seconds. Stir in heavy cream and cheddar and cook until thickened. Add shrimp and coat well. Serve.

Nutrition: Calories: 560 - Fat: 41g - Carbs: 4.3g - Protein: 24.4g.

181.   Grilled Shrimp with Chimichurri Sauce

Preparation time: 10 minutes
Cooking time: 45 minutes
Servings: 4
Ingredients:
- 1lb. shrimp, peeled and deveined
- Olive oil
- Juice of 1 lime

Chimichurri:
- ½ tsp salt
- ¼ cup olive oil
- Garlic cloves
- ¼ cup red onions, chopped
- ¼ cup red wine vinegar
- ½ tsp pepper
- Parsley
- ¼ tsp red pepper flakes

Directions:
1. Process the chimichurri ingredients in a blender until smooth; set aside.
2. Combine shrimp, olive oil, and lime juice, in a bowl, and let marinate in the fridge for 30 minutes.
3. Preheat your grill to medium. Add shrimp and cook about 2 minutes per side. Serve shrimp drizzled with the chimichurri sauce.

Nutrition: Calories: 283 - Fat: 20.3g - Carbs: 3.5g Protein: 16g.

182.   Garlic Parmesan Mahi-Mahi

Preparation Time: 10 minutes
Cooking Time: 10 minutes.
Servings: 2
Ingredients
- 2 fillets of mahi-mahi
- 1 tsp minced garlic
- 1/3 tsp dried thyme
- 1 tbsp. avocado oil
- 1 tbsp. grated parmesan cheese

Seasoning:
- 1/3 tsp salt
- 1/4 tsp ground black pepper

Directions:
1. Turn on the oven, set it to 425°F and let it preheat.
2. Meanwhile, take a small bowl, place oil in it, add garlic, thyme, cheese and oil and stir until mixed.
3. Season fillets with salt and black pepper, then coat with prepared cheese mixture, place fillets in a baking sheet and then cook for 7 to 10 minutes until thoroughly cooked.
4. Serve.

Nutrition: Calories: 170 - Fat: 7.8g - Protein: 22.3g -Carbs: 0.8g - Fibre: 0g.

183. Tilapia with Olives & Tomato Sauce

Preparation time: 5 minutes
Cooking time: 25 minutes
Servings: 4
Ingredients:
- 4 tilapia fillets
- Garlic cloves, minced
- Oregano
- 7oz. diced tomatoes
- 1 tbsp olive oil
- ½ red onion, chopped
- Parsley
- ¼ cup kalamata olives

Directions:
1. Heat olive oil in a skillet over medium heat and cook the onion for 3 minutes.
2. Add garlic and oregano and cook for 40 seconds.
3. Stir in tomatoes and bring the mixture to a boil.
4. Reduce the heat and simmer for 4 minutes.
5. Add olives and tilapia and cook for about 8 minutes.
6. Serve the tilapia with tomato sauce.

Nutrition: Calories: 282 - Fat: 15g - Carbs: 6g - Protein: 23g.

184. Zucchini Noodles in Creamy Salmon Sauce

Preparation Time: 5 minutes.
Cooking Time: 7 minutes.
Servings: 2
Ingredients
- ½ lb. smoked salmon
- 1lb. zucchini, spiralized into noodles
- 1 tbsp. chopped basil
- ½ cup whipping cream
- 2oz. cream cheese, softened
- 1/3 tsp salt
- 1/3 tsp ground black pepper
- 1 tbsp. avocado oil

Directions:
1. Cut zucchini into noodles, place them into a colander, sprinkle with some salt, toss until well coated and set aside for 10 minutes.
2. Meanwhile, take a small saucepan, place it over medium-low heat, add whipped cream in it, add cream cheese, stir until mixed, bring it to a simmer, and cook for 2 minutes or more until smooth.
3. Then switch heat to low heat, add basil into the pan, cut salmon into thin slices, add to the pan, season with ¼ tsp of each salt and black pepper and cook for 1 minute until hot, set aside until required.
4. Take a medium skillet pan, place it over medium-high heat, add oil and when hot, add zucchini noodles and cook for 1 to 2 minutes until fried.
5. Season zucchini with remaining salt and black pepper and then distribute zucchini between two plates.
6. Top zucchini noodles with salmon sauce and then serve.

Nutrition: Calories: 271 - Fat: 22g - Protein: 13.5g - Carbs: 4.5g - Fibre: 1.5g.

185. Roasted Salmon with Kimchi

Preparation time: 10 minutes
Cooking time: 12 minutes
Servings: 2
Ingredients:
- 1 tbsp. ghee, soft
- ½lb. salmon fillets
- 1oz. kimchi, finely chopped
- Salt and black pepper to taste

Directions:
1. In the food processor, mix ghee with kimchi and blend well.
2. Rub salmon with salt, pepper, and Kimchi mix and place into a baking dish.
3. Place in the oven and bake at 420°F for 15 minutes.
4. Serve.

Nutrition: Calories: 200 - Fat: 12g - Carbs: 3g - Protein: 21g.

186.   Lemon Garlic Shrimp

Preparation time: 2 minutes
Cooking time: 20 minutes
Servings: 6
Ingredients:

- ½ cup butter, divided
- 2lb. shrimp, peeled and deveined
- Salt and black pepper to taste
- ¼ tsp sweet paprika
- 1 tbsp minced garlic
- 1 tbsp water
- 1 lemon, zested and juiced
- 1 tbsp chopped parsley

Directions:

1. Melt half of the butter in a large skillet over medium heat, season the shrimp with salt, black pepper, paprika, and add to the butter. Stir in the garlic and cook the shrimp for 4 minutes on both sides until pink. Remove to a bowl and set aside.
2. Put the remaining butter in the skillet; include the lemon zest, juice, and water.
3. Add the shrimp, parsley, and adjust the taste with salt and pepper.
4. Cook for 2 minutes. Serve shrimp and sauce with squash pasta.

Nutrition (per serving): Calories: 258 - Fat: 22g Carbs: 2g - Protein 13g.

187.   Baked Haddock

Preparation time: 10 minutes
Cooking time: 30 minutes
Servings: 2
Ingredients:

- ½ pound haddock
- 1 ½ tsp. water
- 1 tbsp. lemon juice
- Salt and black pepper to taste
- 1 tbsp. mayonnaise
- ½ tsp. dill weed
- Cooking spray
- Pinch of old bay seasoning

Directions:

1. Spray a baking dish with cooking oil.

2. Add lemon juice, water, and fish and toss to coat.
3. Add salt, pepper, old bay seasoning, and dill weed and toss again.
4. Add mayo and spread well.
5. Bake in the oven at 360°F for 30 minutes.
6. Serve.

Nutrition: Calories: 104 - Fat: 12g - Carbs: 0.5g - Protein: 20g.

188.   Trout with Sauce

Preparation time: 1 minutes
Cooking time: 210 minutes
Servings: 2
Ingredients:

- 2 big trout fillets
- Salt and black pepper to taste
- Olive oil
- 1 tbsp. ghee
- Zest and juice from 2 oranges
- Handful parsley, chopped
- 1 cup pecans, chopped

Directions:

1. Heat a pan with oil over medium-high heat.
2. Add the fish fillet and season with salt and pepper.
3. Cook for 4 minutes on each side. Transfer to a plate and keep warm.
4. Heat the same pan with the ghee over medium heat, then add the pecans. Stir and toast for 1 minute.
5. Add orange juice and zest, some salt and pepper and chopped parsley.
6. Stir and cook for 1 minute.
7. Pour the mixture over the fish fillet.
8. Serve.

Nutrition: Calories: 200 - Fat: 10g - Carbs: 1g - Protein: 14g.

Chapter 13. Vegetables

189. Mediterranean Filling Stuffed Portobello Mushrooms

Preparation time: 10 minutes
Cooking time: 35 minutes
Servings: 4
Ingredients:

- Large portobello mushroom caps
- 3 tablespoons good-quality olive oil, divided
- 1 cup chopped fresh spinach
- 1 red bell pepper, chopped
- 1 celery stalk, chopped
- ½ cup chopped sun-dried tomato
- ¼ onion, chopped
- Minced garlic
- 1 teaspoon chopped fresh oregano
- 2 cups chopped pecans
- ¼ cup balsamic vinaigrette
- Sea salt, for seasoning
- Freshly ground black pepper, for seasoning

Directions:

1. Preheat the oven. Set the oven temperature to 350°F. Line a baking sheet with parchment paper.
2. Prepare the mushrooms. Use a spoon to scoop the black gills out of the mushrooms. Massage 2 tablespoons of the olive oil all over the mushroom caps and place the mushrooms on the prepared baking sheet. Set them aside.
3. Prepare the filling. In a large skillet over medium-high heat, warm the remaining 1 tablespoon of olive oil. Add the spinach, red bell pepper, celery, sun-dried tomato, onion, garlic, and oregano and sauté until the vegetables are tender, about 10 minutes. Stir in the pecans and balsamic vinaigrette and season the mixture with salt and pepper.
4. Assemble and bake. Stuff the mushroom caps with the filling and bake for 20 to 25 minutes until they're tender and golden.
5. Serve. Place one stuffed mushroom on each of four plates and serve them hot.

Nutrition: Calories: 595 - Fat: 56g - Fibre: 9g - Carbs: 9g - Sodium: 51mg - Protein: 10g.

190. Pesto-Glazed Cauliflower Steaks with Fresh Basil and Mozzarella

Preparation time: 10 minutes
Cooking time: 20 minutes
Servings: 4
Ingredients:

- Olive oil cooking spray
- 1 head cauliflower, cut into "steaks" about 1 inch thick
- ¼ cup spinach basil pesto
- 1 cup shredded mozzarella cheese
- ¼ cup chopped marinated artichoke hearts
- ¼ cup chopped sun-dried tomatoes
- ¼ cup sliced olives
- Pine nuts

Directions:

1. Preheat the oven. Set the oven temperature to 400°F. Lightly grease a baking sheet with olive oil cooking spray.
2. Assemble the cauliflower steaks. Place the cauliflower steaks in a single layer on the baking sheet and spread 1 tablespoon of pesto on each. Sprinkle with the mozzarella and top with the artichoke hearts, sun-dried tomatoes, olives, and pine nuts.
3. Bake. Bake the cauliflower for 20 minutes until the edges are crispy and the cheese is bubbly and melted.
4. Serve. Divide the cauliflower between four plates and serve it hot.

Nutrition: Calories: 316 - Fat: 23g - Fibre: 6g - Carbs: 8g - Sodium: 465mg - Protein: 14g.

191. Zucchini Roll Manicotti

Preparation time: 15 minutes
Cooking time: 30 minutes
Servings: 4
Ingredients:

- Olive oil cooking spray
- 2lb. zucchini
- Good-quality olive oil
- 1 red bell pepper, diced
- ½ onion, minced
- Minced garlic
- 1 cup goat cheese
- 1 cup shredded mozzarella cheese
- 1 tablespoon chopped fresh oregano
- Sea salt, for seasoning
- Freshly ground black pepper, for seasoning
- 2 cups low-carbs marinara sauce, divided
- ½ cup grated parmesan cheese

Directions:

1. Preheat the oven. Set the oven temperature to 375°F. Lightly grease a 9-by-13-inch baking dish with olive oil cooking spray.
2. Prepare the zucchini. Cut the zucchini lengthwise into ⅛-inch-thick slices and set them aside.
3. Make the filling. In a medium skillet over medium-high heat, warm the olive oil. Add the red bell pepper, onion, and garlic and sauté until they've softened, about 4 minutes. Remove the skillet from the heat and transfer the vegetables to a medium bowl. Stir the goat cheese, mozzarella, and oregano into the vegetables. Season it all with salt and pepper.
4. Assemble the manicotti. Spread 1 cup of the marinara sauce in the bottom of the baking dish. Lay a zucchini slice on a clean cutting board and place a couple tablespoons of filling at one end. Roll the slice up and place it in the baking dish, seam-side down. Repeat with the remaining zucchini slices. Spoon the remaining sauce over the rolls and top with the Parmesan.
5. Bake. Bake the rolls for 30 to 35 minutes until the zucchini is tender and the cheese is golden.
6. Serve. Spoon the rolls onto four plates and serve them hot.

Nutrition: Calories: 342 - Fat: 24g - Fibre: 3g - Carbs: 11g -Sodium: 331mg - Protein: 20g.

192. Zucchini Pasta with Spinach, Olives, And Asiago

Preparation time: 10 minutes
Cooking time: 10 minutes
Servings: 4
Ingredients:

- Good-quality olive oil
- 1 tablespoon grass-fed butter
- 1½ tablespoons minced garlic
- 1 cup packed fresh spinach
- ½ cup sliced black olives
- ½ cup halved cherry tomatoes
- Chopped fresh basil
- 21oz. zucchini, spiralized
- Sea salt, for seasoning
- Freshly ground black pepper, for seasoning
- ½ cup shredded Asiago cheese

Directions:

1. Sauté the vegetables. In a large skillet over medium-high heat, warm the olive oil and butter. Add the garlic and sauté until it's tender, about 2 minutes. Stir in the spinach, olives, tomatoes, and basil and sauté until the spinach is wilted, about 4 minutes. Stir in the zucchini noodles, toss to combine them with the sauce, and cook until the zucchini is tender, about 2 minutes.
2. Serve. Season with salt and pepper. Divide the mixture between four bowls and serve topped with the Asiago.

Nutrition: Calories: 199 - Fat: 18g - Carbs: 3g - Fibre: 1g - Sodium: 363mg - Protein: 6g.

Chapter 13. Vegetables

193. Cheesy Garden Veggie Crustless Quiche

Preparation time: 5 minutes
Cooking time: 25 minutes
Servings: 4
Ingredients:

- 1 tablespoon butter, divided
- 2 eggs
- ¾ cup heavy (whipping) cream
- 3oz. goat cheese, divided
- ½ cup sliced mushrooms, chopped
- 1 scallion, white and green parts, chopped
- 1 cup shredded fresh spinach
- Cherry tomatoes, cut in half

Directions:

1. Preheat the oven. Set the oven temperature to 350°F. Grease a 9-inch pie plate with ½ teaspoon of the butter and set it aside.
2. Mix the quiche base. In a medium bowl, whisk the eggs, cream, and 2 ounces of the cheese until it's all well blended. Set it aside.
3. Sauté the vegetables. In a small skillet over medium-high heat, melt the remaining butter. Add the mushrooms and scallion and sauté them until they've softened, about 2 minutes. Add the spinach and sauté until it's wilted, about 2 minutes.
4. Assemble and bake. Spread the vegetable mixture in the bottom of the pie plate and pour the egg-and-cream mixture over the vegetables. Scatter the cherry tomatoes and the remaining 1 ounce of goat cheese on top. Bake for 20 to 25 minutes until the quiche is cooked through, puffed, and lightly browned.
5. Serve. Cut the quiche into wedges and divide it between four plates. Serve it warm or cold.

Nutrition: Calories: 355 - Fat: 30g - Carbs: 4g - Fibre: 1g - Sodium: 228mg - Protein: 18g.

194. Spinach Artichoke Stuffed Peppers

Preparation time: 10 minutes
Cooking time: 20 minutes
Servings: 4
Ingredients:

- 4 red bell peppers, halved and seeded
- Good-quality olive oil, for drizzling
- Sea salt, for seasoning
- Freshly ground black pepper, for seasoning
- 2 cups finely chopped cauliflower
- 10oz. chopped fresh spinach
- 1 (14-oz.) can artichoke hearts, drained and chopped
- 1 cup cream cheese, softened
- 1½ cups shredded mozzarella cheese, divided
- ½ cup sour cream
- ¼ cup mayonnaise
- 2 teaspoons minced garlic

Directions:

1. Preheat the oven. Set the oven temperature to 400°F. Line a baking sheet with parchment paper.
2. Prepare the peppers. Place the red bell peppers cut side up on the baking sheet. Lightly grease them all over with the olive oil and season them with salt and pepper.
3. Make the filling. In a large bowl, mix together the cauliflower, spinach, artichoke hearts, cream cheese, ¾ cup of the mozzarella, and the sour cream, mayonnaise, and garlic.
4. Stuff and bake. Stuff the peppers with the filling and sprinkle with the remaining ¾ cup of mozzarella. Bake them for 20 to 25 minutes until the filling is heated through, bubbly, and lightly browned.
5. Serve. Place one stuffed pepper on each of four plates and serve them hot.

Nutrition: Calories: 523 - Fat: 43g - Fibre: 7g - Carbs: 12g - Sodium: 355mg - Protein: 19g.

195. Turnip Greens with Sausage

Preparation time: 2 minutes
Cooking time: 8 minutes
Servings: 4
Ingredients:

- Sesame oil
- 1lb. pork sausages, casing removed sliced
- garlic cloves, minced
- 1 medium-sized leek, chopped
- 1lb. turnip greens
- 1 cup turkey bone stock
- Sea salt, to taste
- 1/4 teaspoon ground black pepper, or more to taste
- 1 bay leaf
- 1 tablespoon black sesame seeds

Directions:

1. Press the "Sauté" button to heat up the Instant Pot. Then, heat the sesame oil; cook the sausage until nice and delicately browned; set aside.
2. Add the garlic and leeks; continue to cook in pan drippings for a minute or two.
3. Add the greens, stock, salt, black pepper, and bay leaf.
4. Secure the lid. Choose "Manual" mode and Low pressure; cook for 3 minutes. Once cooking is complete, use a quick pressure release; carefully remove the lid.
5. Serve garnished with black sesame seeds and enjoy!

Nutrition: Calories: 149 - Fat: 7.2g - Carbs: 9g - Protein: 14.2g - Sugars: 2.2g.

196. Vegetable Vodka Sauce Bake

Preparation time: 10 minutes
Cooking time: 30 minutes
Servings: 4
Ingredients:

- 3 tablespoons melted butter, divided
- 2 cups mushrooms, halved
- 2 cups cooked cauliflower florets
- 1½ cups purchased vodka sauce
- ¾ cup heavy (whipping) cream
- ½ cup grated asiago cheese
- Sea salt, for seasoning
- Freshly ground black pepper, for seasoning
- 1 cup shredded provolone cheese
- Chopped fresh oregano

Directions:

1. Preheat the oven. Set the oven temperature to 350°F and use 1 tablespoon of the melted butter to grease a 9-by-13-inch baking dish.
2. Mix the vegetables. In a large bowl, combine the mushrooms, cauliflower, vodka sauce, cream, Asiago, and the remaining 2 tablespoons of butter. Season the vegetables with salt and pepper.
3. Bake. Transfer the vegetable mixture to the baking dish and top it with the provolone cheese. Bake for 30 to 35 minutes until it's bubbly and heated through.
4. Serve. Divide the mixture between four plates and top with the oregano.

Nutrition: Calories: 537 - Fat: 45g - Fibre: 6g - Carbs: 8g - Sodium: 527mg - Protein: 19g.

197. Easy Cheesy Artichokes

Preparation time: 5 minutes
Cooking time: 5 minutes
Servings: 3
Ingredients:

- Medium-sized artichokes, cleaned and trimmed
- Cloves garlic, smashed
- 2 tablespoons butter, melted
- Sea salt, to taste
- 1/2 teaspoon cayenne pepper
- 1/4 teaspoon ground black pepper, or more to taste
- 1 lemon, freshly squeezed
- 1 cup monterey-jack cheese, shredded
- 1 tablespoon fresh parsley, roughly chopped

Directions:

1. Start by adding 1 cup of water and a steamer basket to the Instant Pot. Place the artichokes in the steamer basket; add garlic and butter.
2. Secure the lid. Choose "Manual" mode and High pressure; cook for 8 minutes. Once cooking is complete, use a quick pressure release; carefully remove the lid.
3. Season your artichokes with salt, cayenne pepper, and black pepper. Now, drizzle them with lemon j   juice.
4. Top with cheese and parsley and serve immediately.

Nutrition: Calories: 173 - Fat: 12.5g - Carbs: 9g Protein: 8.1g - Sugars: 0.9g.

198. Chinese Bok Choy

Preparation time: 2 minutes
Cooking time: 8 minutes
Servings: 4
Ingredients:

- Butter, melted
- Cloves garlic, minced
- 1 (1/2-inch) slice fresh ginger root, grated
- 1 ½lb. bok choy, trimmed
- 1 cup vegetable stock
- Celery salt and ground black pepper to taste
- 1 teaspoon five-spice powder
- Soy sauce

Directions:

1. Press the "Sauté" button to heat up the Instant Pot. Now, warm the butter and sauté the garlic until tender and fragrant.
2. Now, add grated ginger and cook for a further 40 seconds.
3. Add Bok choy, stock, salt, black pepper, and Five-spice powder.
4. Secure the lid. Choose "Manual" mode and High pressure; cook for 6 minutes. Once cooking is complete, use a quick pressure release; carefully remove the lid.
5. Drizzle soy sauce over your Bok choy and serve immediately.

Nutrition: Calories: 83 - Fat: 6.1g - Carbs: 5.7g - Protein: 3.2g - Sugars: 2.4g.

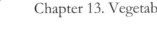

199. Green Cabbage with Bacon

Preparation time: 2 minutes
Cooking time: 8 minutes
Servings: 4
Ingredients:

- Olive oil
- 4 slices bacon, chopped
- 1 head green cabbage, cored and cut into wedges
- 2 cups vegetable stock
- Sea salt, to taste
- 1/2 teaspoon whole black peppercorns
- 1 teaspoon cayenne pepper
- 1 bay leaf

Directions:

1. Press the "Sauté" button to heat up the Instant Pot. Then, heat olive oil and cook the bacon until it is nice and delicately browned.
2. Then, add the remaining ingredients; gently stir to combine.
3. Secure the lid. Choose "Manual" mode and High pressure; cook for 3 minutes. Once cooking is complete, use a quick pressure release; carefully remove the lid.
4. Serve warm and enjoy!

Nutrition: Calories: 166 - Fat: 13g - Carbs: 7.1g - Protein: 6.8g - Sugars: 2.7g.

200. Warm Broccoli Salad Bowl

Preparation time: 2 minutes
Cooking time: 8 minutes
Servings: 4
Ingredients:

- 1lb. broccoli, broken into florets
- Balsamic vinegar
- Garlic cloves, minced
- 1 teaspoon mustard seeds
- 1 teaspoon cumin seeds
- Salt and pepper, to taste
- 1 cup Cottage cheese, crumbled

Directions:

1. Place 1 cup of water and a steamer basket in your Instant Pot.
2. Place the broccoli in the steamer basket.

3. Secure the lid. Choose "Manual" mode and High pressure; cook for 5 minutes. Once cooking is complete, use a quick pressure release; carefully remove the lid.
4. Then, toss your broccoli with the other ingredients. Serve and enjoy!

Nutrition: Calories: 95 - Fat: 3.1g - Carbs: 8.1g - Protein: 9.9g - Sugars: 3.8g.

201. Creamed Spinach with Cheese

Preparation time: 2 minutes
Cooking time: 8 minutes
Servings: 4
Ingredients:

- 2 tablespoons butter, melted
- 1/2 cup scallions, chopped
- Cloves garlic, smashed
- 1 ½lb. fresh spinach
- 1 cup vegetable broth, preferably homemade
- 1 cup cream cheese, cubed
- Seasoned salt and ground black pepper, to taste
- 1/2 teaspoon dried dill weed

Directions:

1. Press the "Sauté" button to heat up the Instant Pot. Then, melt the butter; cook the scallions and garlic until tender and aromatic.
2. Add the remaining ingredients and stir to combine well.
3. Secure the lid. Choose "Manual" mode and High pressure; cook for 2 minutes. Once cooking is complete, use a quick pressure release; carefully remove the lid.
4. Ladle into individual bowls and serve warm.

Nutrition: Calories: 283 - Fat: 23.9g - Carbs: 9g - Protein: 10.7g -Sugars: 3.2g.

202. Asparagus with Colby Cheese

Preparation time: 2 minutes
Cooking time: 8 minutes
Servings: 4
Ingredients:

- 1 ½ pounds fresh asparagus
- Olive oil
- Garlic cloves, minced
- Sea salt, to taste
- 1/4 teaspoon ground black pepper
- 1/2 cup Colby cheese, shredded

Directions:

1. Add 1 cup of water and a steamer basket to your Instant Pot.
2. Now, place the asparagus on the steamer basket; drizzle your asparagus with olive oil. Scatter garlic over the top of the asparagus.
3. Season with salt and black pepper.
4. Secure the lid. Choose "Manual" mode and High pressure; cook for 1 minute. Once cooking is complete, use a quick pressure release; carefully remove the lid.
5. Transfer the prepared asparagus to a nice serving platter and scatter shredded cheese over the top. Enjoy!

Nutrition: Calories: 12.2 - Fat: 164g - Carbs: 8.1g Protein: 7.8g - Sugars: 3.3g.

203. Mediterranean Aromatic Zucchini

Preparation time: 2 minutes
Cooking time: 8 minutes
Servings: 4
Ingredients:

- Olive oil
- Garlic cloves, chopped
- 1lb. zucchini, sliced
- 1/2 cup tomato purée
- 1/2 cup water
- 1 teaspoon dried thyme
- 1/2 teaspoon dried oregano
- 1/2 teaspoon dried rosemary

Directions:

1. Press the "Sauté" button to heat up the Instant Pot. Then, heat the olive oil; sauté the garlic until aromatic.
2. Add the remaining ingredients.
3. Secure the lid. Choose "Manual" mode and Low pressure; cook for 3 minutes. Once cooking is complete, use a quick pressure release; carefully remove the lid.

Nutrition: Calories: 85 - Fat: 7.1g - Carbs: 4.7g - Protein: 1.6g - Sugars: 3.3g.

204. Family Cauliflower Soup

Preparation time: 2 minutes
Cooking time: 8 minutes
Servings: 4
Ingredients:

- Butter, softened
- 1/2 cup leeks, thinly sliced
- Cloves garlic, minced
- 3/4lb. cauliflower, broken into florets
- 1 cup water
- 2 cups chicken stock
- 1 cup full-fat milk
- Kosher salt, to taste
- 1/3 teaspoon ground black pepper

Directions:

1. Press the "Sauté" button to heat up your Instant Pot. Then, melt the butter; sauté the leeks until softened.
2. Then, sauté the garlic until fragrant, about 30 seconds. Add the remaining ingredients and gently stir to combine.
3. Secure the lid. Choose "Manual" mode and Low pressure; cook for 5 minutes. Once cooking is complete, use a quick pressure release; carefully remove the lid.
4. Ladle into individual bowls and serve warm.

Nutrition: Calories: 167 - Fat: 13.7g - Carbs: 8.7g Protein: 3.8g - Sugars: 5.1g.

205. Chanterelles with Cheddar Cheese

Preparation time: 2 minutes
Cooking time: 8 minutes
Servings: 4
Ingredients:
- 1 tablespoon olive oil
- Cloves garlic, minced
- 1 (1-inch) ginger root, grated
- 1/2 teaspoon dried dill weed
- 1 teaspoon dried basil
- 1/2 teaspoon dried thyme
- 12oz. chanterelle mushrooms, clean and sliced
- 1/2 cup water
- 1/2 cup tomato purée
- 2 tablespoons dry white wine
- 1/3 teaspoon freshly ground black pepper
- Kosher salt, to taste
- 1 cup cheddar cheese

Directions:
1. Press the "Sauté" button to heat up the Instant Pot. Then, heat the olive oil; sauté the garlic and grated ginger for 1 minute or until aromatic.
2. Add dried dill, basil, thyme, Chanterelles, water, tomato purée, dry white wine, black pepper, and salt.
3. Secure the lid. Choose "Manual" mode and Low pressure; cook for 5 minutes. Once cooking is complete, use a quick pressure release; carefully remove the lid.
4. Top with shredded cheese and serve immediately.

Nutrition: Calories: 218 - Fat: 15.1g - Carbs: 9.5g Protein: 9.9g - Sugars: 2.3g.

206. Cauliflower and Kohlrabi Mash

Preparation time: 2 minutes
Cooking time: 15 minutes
Servings: 4
Ingredients:
- ½ lb. cauliflower, cut into florets
- ½ lb. kohlrabi, peeled and diced
- 1 cup water
- 3/4 cup sour cream
- 1 garlic clove, minced
- Sea salt, to taste
- 1/3 teaspoon ground black pepper
- 1/2 teaspoon cayenne pepper

Directions:
1. Add 1 cup of water and a steamer basket to the bottom of your Instant Pot.
2. Then, arrange cauliflower and kohlrabi in the steamer basket.
3. Secure the lid. Choose "Manual" mode and Low pressure; cook for 3 minutes. Once cooking is complete, use a quick pressure release; carefully remove the lid.
4. Now, puree the cauliflower and kohlrabi with a potato masher. Add the remaining ingredients and stir well.

Nutrition: Calories: 89 - Fat: 4.7g - Carbs: 9.6g - Protein: 3.6g - Sugars: 2.6g.

207. Bell Pepper Eggs

Preparation time: 10 minutes
Cooking time: 4 minutes
Servings: 2
Ingredients:
- 1 green bell pepper,
- Eggs

Seasoning:
- 1 tsp coconut oil
- ¼ tsp salt
- ¼ tsp ground black pepper

Directions:
1. Prepare pepper rings, and for this, cut out two slices from the pepper, about ¼-inch, and reserve remaining bell pepper for later use.
2. Take a skillet pan, place it over medium heat, grease it with oil, place pepper rings in it, and then crack an egg into each ring.
3. Season eggs with salt and black pepper, cook for 4 minutes or until eggs have cooked to the desired level.
4. Transfer eggs to a plate and serve.

Nutrition: Calories: 110 - Fat: 8g - Protein: 7.2g Carbs: 1.7g - Fibre: 1.1g.

208.   Buttery and Garlicky Fennel

Preparation time: 2 minutes
Cooking time: 6 minutes
Servings: 6
Ingredients:

- 1/2 stick butter
- Garlic cloves, sliced
- 1/2 teaspoon sea salt
- 1 ½ pounds fennel bulbs, cut into wedges
- 1/4 teaspoon ground black pepper, or more to taste
- 1/2 teaspoon cayenne pepper
- 1/4 teaspoon dried dill weed
- 1/3 cup dry white wine
- 2/3 cup chicken stock

Directions:

1. Press the "Sauté" button to heat up your Instant Pot; now, melt the butter. Cook garlic for 30 seconds, stirring periodically.
2. Add the remaining ingredients.
3. Secure the lid. Choose "Manual" mode and Low pressure; cook for 3 minutes. Once cooking is complete, use a quick pressure release; carefully remove the lid.

Nutrition: Calories: 111- Fat: 7.8g - Carbs: 8.7g - Protein: 2.1g- Sugars: 4.7g.

209.   Cabbage Hash Browns

Preparation time: 10 minutes.
Cooking time: 12 minutes
Servings: 2
Ingredients:

- 1 ½ cup shredded cabbage
- Slices of bacon
- 1/2 tsp garlic powder
- 1 egg

Seasoning:

- 1 tbsp coconut oil
- ½ tsp salt
- 1/8 tsp ground black pepper

Directions:

1. Crack the egg in a bowl, add garlic powder, black pepper, and salt, whisk well, then add cabbage, toss until well mixed and shape the mixture into four patties.
2. Take a large skillet pan, place it over medium heat, add oil and when hot, add patties in it and cook for 3 minutes per side until golden brown.
3. Transfer hash browns to a plate, then add bacon into the pan and cook for 5 minutes until crispy.
4. Serve hash browns with bacon.

Nutrition: Calories: 336 - Fat: 29.5g - Protein: 16g - Carbs: 0.9g - Fibre: 0.8g.

210.   Omelet-Stuffed Peppers

Preparation time: 5 minutes
Cooking time: 20 minutes
Servings: 2
Ingredients:

- 1 large green bell pepper, halved, cored
- 2 eggs
- 1 slices of bacon, chopped, cooked
- 1 tbsp grated parmesan cheese

Seasoning:

- 1/3 tsp salt
- ¼ tsp ground black pepper

Directions:

1. Turn on the oven, then set it to 400°F, and let preheat.
2. Then take a baking dish, pour in 1 tbsp water, place bell pepper halved in it, cut side up, and bake for 5 minutes.
3. Meanwhile, crack eggs in a bowl, add chopped bacon and cheese, season with salt and black pepper, and whisk until combined.
4. After 5 minutes of baking time, remove baking dish from the oven, evenly fill the peppers with egg mixture and continue baking for 15 to 20 minutes until eggs has set.
5. Serve.

Nutrition: Calories: 428 - Fat: 35.2g - Protein: 23.5g - Carbs: 2.8g - Fibre: 1.5g.

211.   Vegetables à la Grecque

Preparation time: 2 minutes
Cooking time: 8 minutes
Servings: 4
Ingredients:
- Olive oil
- Garlic cloves, minced
- 1 red onion, chopped
- 14oz. button mushrooms, thinly sliced
- 1 (1-pound) eggplant, sliced
- 1/2 teaspoon dried basil
- 1 teaspoon dried oregano
- 1 thyme sprig, leaves picked
- Rosemary sprigs, leaves picked
- 1/2 cup tomato sauce
- 1/4 cup dry Greek wine
- 1/4 cup water
- 7oz. halloumi cheese, cubed
- Kalamata olives, pitted and halved

Directions:
1. Press the "Sauté" button to heat up your Instant Pot; now, heat the olive oil. Cook the garlic and red onions for 1 to 2 minutes, stirring periodically.
2. Stir in the mushrooms and continue to sauté an additional 2 to 3 minutes.
3. Add the eggplant, basil, oregano, thyme, rosemary, tomato sauce, Greek wine, and water.
4. Secure the lid. Choose "Manual" mode and Low pressure; cook for 3 minutes. Once cooking is complete, use a quick pressure release; carefully remove the lid.
5. Top with cheese and olives.

Nutrition: Calories: 326 - Fat: 25.1g - Carbs: 8.4g Protein: 15.7g - Sugars: 4.3g.

212.   Cauliflower Hash Browns

Preparation time: 10 minutes
Cooking time: 18 minutes
Servings: 2
Ingredients
- ¾ cup grated cauliflower
- Slices of bacon
- 1/2 tsp garlic powder
- 1 large egg white

Seasoning:
- 1 tbsp coconut oil
- ½ tsp salt
- 1/8 tsp ground black pepper

Directions:
1. Place grated cauliflower in a heatproof bowl, cover with plastic wrap, poke some holes in it with a fork and then microwave for 3 minutes until tender.
2. Let steamed cauliflower cool for 10 minutes, then wrap in a cheesecloth and squeeze well to drain moisture as much as possible.
3. Crack the egg in a bowl, add garlic powder, black pepper, and salt, whisk well, then add cauliflower, and toss until well mixed and sticky mixture comes together.
4. Take a large skillet pan, place it over medium heat, add oil and when hot, drop cauliflower mixture on it, press lightly to form hash brown patties, and cook for 3 to 4 minutes per side until browned.
5. Transfer hash browns to a plate, then add bacon into the pan and cook for 5 minutes until crispy.
6. Serve hash browns with bacon.

Nutrition: Calories: 348 - Fat: 31g - Carbs:1.2g - Protein: 15.6g - Fibre: 0.5g.

213.   Egg in a Hole with Eggplant

Preparation time: 5 minutes
Cooking time: 15 minutes
Servings: 2
Ingredients:

- 1 large eggplant
- Eggs
- 1 tbsp coconut oil, melted
- 1 tsp unsalted butter
- 1 tbsp chopped green onions

Seasoning:

- ¾ tsp ground black pepper
- ¾ tsp salt

Directions:

1. Set the grill and let it preheat at the high setting.
2. Meanwhile, prepare the eggplant, and for this, cut two slices from eggplant, about 1-inch thick, and reserve the remaining eggplant for later use.
3. Brush slices of eggplant with oil, season with salt on both sides, then place the slices on grill and cook for 3 to 4 minutes per side.
4. Transfer grilled eggplant to a cutting board, let it cool for 5 minutes and then make a home in the center of each slice by using a cookie cutter.
5. Take a frying pan, place it over medium heat, add butter and when it melts, add eggplant slices in it and crack an egg into its each hole.
6. Let the eggs cook for 3 to 4 minutes, then carefully flip the eggplant slice and continue cooking for 3 minutes until the egg has thoroughly cooked.
7. Season egg with salt and black pepper, transfer them to a plate, then garnish with green onions and serve.

Nutrition: Calories: 184 - Fat: 14.1g - Carbs: 3g - Protein: 7.8g - Fibre: 3.5g.

214.   Breakfast Burgers with Avocado

Preparation time: 5 minutes
Cooking time: 15 minutes
Servings: 2
Ingredients:

- 4 strips of bacon
- 2 tablespoons of chopped lettuce
- 2 avocados
- 2 eggs
- Mayonnaise

Seasoning:

- ¼ tsp salt
- ¼ tsp sesame seeds

Directions:

1. Take a skillet pan, place it over medium heat and when hot, add bacon strips and cook for 5 minutes until crispy.
2. Transfer bacon to a plate lined with paper towels, crack an egg into the pan, and cook for 2 to 4 minutes or until fried to the desired level; fry remaining egg in the same manner.
3. Prepare sandwiches and for this, cut each avocado in half widthwise, remove the pit, and scoop out the flesh.
4. Fill the hollow of two avocado halves with mayonnaise, then top each half with 1 tbsp of chopped lettuce, 2 bacon strips, and a fried egg, and then cover with the second half of avocado.
5. Sprinkle sesame seeds on avocados and serve.

Nutrition: Calories: 205 - Fat: 18.5g - Carbs: 0.7g Protein: 7.7g - Fibre: 1.9g.

215.   Bacon Avocado Bombs

Preparation time: 10 minutes
Cooking time: 10 minutes
Servings: 2
Ingredients:
- 1 avocado, halved, pitted
- Slices of bacon
- 1 tbsp grated parmesan cheese

Directions:
1. Turn on the oven and broiler and let it preheat.
2. Meanwhile, prepare the avocado and for that, cut it in half, then remove its pit, and then peel the skin.
3. Evenly one half of the avocado with cheese, replace with the other half of avocado and then wrap avocado with bacon slices.
4. Take a baking sheet, line it with aluminum foil, place wrapped avocado on it, and broil for 5 minutes per side, flipping carefully with tong halfway.
5. When done, cut each avocado in half crosswise and serve.

Nutrition: Calories: 378 - Fat: 33.6g - Carbs: 0.5g Protein: 15g - Fibre: 2.3g.

216.   Frittata with Spinach and Meat

Preparation time: 10 minutes
Cooking time: 20 minutes
Servings: 2
Ingredients:
- 9oz. ground turkey
- 9oz. of spinach leaves
- 1/3 tsp minced garlic
- 1/3 tsp coconut oil
- 2 eggs

Seasoning:
- 1/3 tsp salt
- ¼ tsp ground black pepper

Directions:
1. Turn on the oven, then set it to 400°F, and let it preheat.
2. Meanwhile, take a skillet pan, place it over medium heat, add spinach and cook

for 3 to 5 minutes until spinach leaves have wilted, remove the pan from heat.
3. Take a small heatproof skillet pan, place it over medium heat, add ground turkey and cook for 5 minutes until thoroughly cooked.
4. Then add spinach, season with salt and black pepper, stir well, then remove the pan from heat and spread the mixture evenly in the pan.
5. Crack eggs in a bowl, season with salt and black pepper, then pour this mixture over spinach mixture in the pan and bake for 10 to 15 minutes until frittata has thoroughly cooked and the top is golden brown.
6. When done, let frittata rest in the pan for 5 minutes, then cut it into slices and serve.

Nutrition: Calories: 166 - Fat: 13g - Protein: 10g Carbs: 0.5g - Fibre: 0.5g.

217.   Spinach and Eggs Scramble

Preparation time: 5 minutes
Cooking time: 10 minutes
Servings: 2
Ingredients:
- 7oz. spinach
- ¼ tsp salt
- 1/8 tsp ground black pepper
- 1 tbsp unsalted butter
- 2 eggs, beaten

Directions:
1. Take a frying pan, place it over medium heat, add butter and when it melts, add spinach and cook for 5 minutes until leaves have wilted.
2. Then pour in eggs, season with salt and black pepper, and cook for 3 minutes until eggs have scramble to the desired level.
3. Serve.

Nutrition: Calories: 90 - Fat: 7g - Protein: 5.6g - Carbs: 0.7g - Fibre: 0.6g.

218. Avocado Egg Boat with Cheddar

Preparation time: 5 minutes
Cooking time: 15 minutes
Servings: 2
Ingredients:

- 1 avocado, halved, pitted
- 2 eggs
- 1 tbsp chopped bacon
- 1 tbsp shredded cheddar cheese

Seasoning:

- 1/8 tsp salt
- 1/8 tsp ground black pepper

Directions:

1. Turn on the oven, then set it to 400°F and let it preheat.
2. Meanwhile, prepare avocado and for this, cut it into half lengthwise and then remove the pit.
3. Scoop out some of the flesh from the center, crack an egg into each half, then sprinkle with bacon and season with salt and black pepper.
4. Sprinkle cheese over egg and avocado and then bake for 10 to 15 minutes or until the yolk has cooked to desired level.
5. Serve.

Nutrition: Calories: 263.5 - Fat: 21.4g - Protein: 12g - Carbs: 1.3g – Fibre: 4.6g.

219. Brussel Sprouts Bacon Breakfast Hash

Preparation time: 5 minutes
Cooking time: 25 minutes
Servings: 2
Ingredients:

- 9oz. brussel sprouts, sliced
- Slices of bacon, chopped
- ½ tsp minced garlic
- ¾ tbsp apple cider vinegar
- 1 egg

Directions:

1. Place a skillet pan over medium heat and when hot, add bacon and cook for 5 to 7 minutes until crispy.
2. Transfer bacon to a plate, add garlic and cook for 30 seconds until fragrant.

3. Then add Brussel sprouts, stir in vinegar and cook for 5 minutes until tender.
4. Return bacon into the pan, cook for 5 minutes until sprouts are golden brown, then create a well in the pan and cracks the egg in it.
5. Cook the eggs for 3 to 5 minutes until cooked to the desired level and then serve immediately.

Nutrition: Calories: 134.5 - Fat: 8.2g - Protein: 10.8g - Carbs: 2.8g - Fibre: 1.6g.

220. Cauliflower and Bacon Hash

Preparation time: 5 minutes
Cooking time: 15 minutes
Servings: 2
Ingredients:

- ½ cup chopped cauliflower florets
- 4 slices of bacon, diced
- ¼ tsp paprika
- 1 tbsp avocado oil

Seasoning:

- 1/3 tsp salt
- 1/8 tsp ground black pepper
- 1 ½ tbsp water

Directions:

1. Take a skillet pan, place it over medium-high heat, add bacon, and cook for 3 to 5 minutes until crispy.
2. Transfer bacon to a plate, then add cauliflower into the pan and cook for 3 minutes until golden.
3. Season with salt, black pepper, and paprika, drizzle with water, and cook for 3 to 5 minutes until cauliflower has softened.
4. Chop the bacon, add it into the pan, stir well, cook for 2 minutes and then remove the pan from heat.
5. Serve.

Nutrition: Calories: 211.5 - Fat: 18.6g - Protein: 9g - Carbs: 1.3g - Fibre: 0.3g.

221.   Vegetable Greek Moussaka

Preparation Time: 10 minutes
Cooking Time: 40 minutes
Servings: 6
Ingredients:

- Large eggplants, cut into strips
- 1 cup diced celery
- 1 cup diced carrots
- 1 small white onion, chopped
- 2 eggs
- 1 tsp olive oil
- 2 cups grated Parmesan
- 1 cup ricotta cheese
- Cloves garlic, minced
- 1 tsp Italian seasoning blend
- Salt to taste

Sauce:

- 1 ½ cups heavy cream
- ¼ cup butter, melted
- 1 cup grated mozzarella cheese
- 1 tsp Italian seasoning
- ¾ cup almond flour

Directions:

1. Preheat the oven to 350°F. Put the eggplant strips on a paper towel, sprinkle with salt, and let sit there to exude liquid. Heat olive oil in a skillet over medium heat and sauté the onion, celery, and carrots for 5 minutes. Stir in the garlic and cook further for 30 seconds; set aside to cool.
2. Mix the eggs, 1 cup of Parmesan cheese, ricotta cheese, and salt in a bowl; set aside. Pour the heavy cream in a pot and bring to heat over a medium fire while continually stirring. Stir in the remaining Parmesan cheese, and 1 teaspoon of Italian seasoning. Turn the heat off and set aside.
3. To lay the moussaka, spread a small amount of the sauce at the bottom of the baking dish. Pat dry the eggplant strips and make a single layer on the sauce. Put a layer of ricotta cheese on the eggplants, sprinkle some veggies on it, and repeat the layering process until all the ingredients are exhausted.
4. In a small bowl, evenly mix the melted butter, almond flour, and 1 teaspoon of Italian seasoning. Spread the top of the moussaka layers with it and sprinkle the top with mozzarella cheese. Cover the dish using foil and place it in the oven to bake for 25 minutes. Take off the foil then bake for at least 5 minutes until the cheese is slightly burned. Slice the moussaka and serve warm.

Nutrition: Calories: 476 - Fat: 35g - Carbs: 9.6g - Protein: 33g.

222.   Zucchini and Broccoli Fritters

Preparation time: 10 minutes
Cooking time: 10 minutes
Servings: 2
Ingredients:

- 1 ounce chopped broccoli
- 1 zucchini, grated, squeezed
- 2 eggs
- 1 tbsp almond flour
- ½ tsp nutritional yeast

Seasoning:

- 1/3 tsp salt
- ¼ tsp dried basil
- 1 tbsp avocado oil

Directions:

1. Wrap grated zucchini in a cheesecloth, twist it well to remove excess moisture, and then place zucchini in a bowl.
2. Add remaining Ingredients, except for oil, and then whisk well until combined.
3. Take a skillet pan, place it over medium heat, add oil and when hot, drop zucchini mixture in four portions, shape them into flat patties and cook for 4 minutes per side until thoroughly cooked.
4. Serve.

Nutrition: Calories: 191 - Fat: 16.6g - Protein: 9.6g - Carbs: 0.8g - Fibre: 0.2g.

223.   Bacon and Avocado Salad

Preparation time: 5 minutes
Cooking time: 8 minutes
Servings: 2
Ingredients:
- 4 slices of bacon, chopped
- 7oz. chopped lettuce
- ½ of a medium avocado, sliced
- 1 tbsp avocado oil
- 1 tbsp apple cider vinegar

Directions:
1. Prepare bacon and for this, place a skillet pan over medium heat and when hot, add chopped bacon and cook for 5 to 8 minutes until golden brown.
2. Then distribute lettuce and avocado between two plates, top with bacon, drizzle with avocado oil and apple cider and serve.

Nutrition: Calories: 147.6 - Fat: 13.6g - Protein: 6g - Carbs: 1.7g - Fibre: 0.6g.

224.   Vegetable Tempeh Kabobs

Preparation Time: 10 minutes
Cooking Time: 16 minutes
Servings: 2
Ingredients:
- 7oz. tempeh, cut into chunks
- 1 ½ cups water
- 1 red onion, cut into chunks
- 1 red bell pepper, cut chunks
- 1 yellow bell pepper, cut into chunks
- Olive oil
- 1 cup sugar-free barbecue sauce

Directions:
1. Place the water to boil in a pot over medium heat, and once it has boiled, turn the heat off, and add the tempeh. Cover the pot and let the tempeh steam for 5 minutes to remove its bitterness.
2. Drain the tempeh after. Pour the barbecue sauce in a bowl, add the tempeh to it, and coat with the sauce. Cover the bowl then marinate in the fridge for 2 hours.
3. Preheat grill to 350ºF, and thread the tempeh, yellow bell pepper, red bell pepper, and onion.
4. Brush the grate of the grill with olive oil, place the skewers on it, and brush with barbecue sauce. Cook the kabobs for 3 minutes on each side while rotating and brushing with more barbecue sauce.
5. Once ready, transfer the kabobs to a plate and serve with lemon cauli couscous and a tomato sauce.

Nutrition: Calories: 228 - Fat: 15g - Carbs: 3.6g - Protein: 13.2g.

225.   Parmesan Roasted Cabbage

Preparation Time: 5 minutes
Cooking Time: 20 minutes
Servings: 4
Ingredients:
- 1 large head green cabbage
- 1 tbsp. melted butter
- 1 tsp garlic powder
- Salt and black pepper to taste
- 1 cup grated Parmesan cheese
- Grated parmesan cheese for topping
- 1 tbsp. chopped parsley to garnish

Directions:
1. Set the oven to 400°F, line baking sheet using foil, and grease with cooking spray.
2. Stand the cabbage and run a knife from the top to bottom to cut the cabbage into wedges. Remove stems and wilted leaves. Mix the butter, garlic, salt, and black pepper until evenly combined.
3. Brush the mixture every side of the cabbage wedges and sprinkle with Parmesan cheese.
4. Put on the baking sheet, then bake for at least 20 minutes to soften the cabbage and melt the cheese. Remove the cabbages when golden brown, plate, and sprinkle with extra cheese and parsley. Serve warm with pan-glazed tofu.

Nutrition: Calories: 268 - Fat: 19.3g - Carbs: 4g - Protein: 17.5g.

226. Asparagus and Tarragon Flan

Preparation Time: 10 minutes
Cooking Time: 55 minutes
Servings: 4
Ingredients:

- 16 asparagus, stems trimmed
- 1 cup water
- ½ cup whipping cream
- 1 cup almond milk
- 2 eggs + 2 egg yolks, beaten in a bowl
- 1 tbsp. chopped tarragon, fresh
- Salt and black pepper to taste
- A small pinch of nutmeg
- 1 tbsp. grated Parmesan cheese
- 3 cups water
- 1 tbsp. butter, melted
- 1 tbsp. butter, softened

Directions:

1. Pour the water and some salt in a pot, add the asparagus, and bring them to boil over medium heat on a stovetop for 6 minutes. Drain the asparagus; cut their tips, and reserve for garnishing. Chop the remaining asparagus into small pieces.

2. In a blender, add the chopped asparagus, whipping cream, almond milk, tarragon, ½ teaspoon of salt, nutmeg, pepper, and Parmesan cheese. Process the ingredients on high speed until smooth. Pour the mixture through a sieve into a bowl and whisk the eggs into it.

3. Preheat the oven to 350ºF. Grease the ramekins with softened butter and share the asparagus mixture among the ramekins. Pour the melted butter over each mixture and top with 2-3 asparagus tips. Pour the remaining water into a baking dish, place it in the ramekins, and insert it in the oven.

4. Bake for 45 minutes until their middle parts are no longer watery. Remove the ramekins and let cool. Garnish the flan with the asparagus tips and serve with chilled white wine.

Nutrition: Calories: 264 - Fat: 11.6g - Carbs: 2.5g Protein: 12.5g.

Chapter 14. Snacks

227.   Crispy Bacon Fat Bombs

Preparation time: 10 minutes
Cooking time: 3 minutes
Servings: 4
Ingredients:

- 2 thick bacon slices (6inch long)
- ½ cup cream cheese
- 1 green chilli, seeded, chopped
- 1 tsp onion powder
- Salt and pepper to taste

Directions:

1. Cook the bacon in a skillet for 3 minutes. Let cool, then crumble. Reserve the bacon fat.
2. In a bowl, combine the remaining ingredients. Add the bacon fat and mix.
3. Shape the mixture into 4 fat bombs. Refrigerate for 30 min.
4. Roll the fat bombs in the crumbled bacon. Serve.

Nutrition: Calories: 141 - Carbs: 0.5g - Fat: 12.9g Protein: 5.7g.

228.   Raspberry Cream Fat Bombs

Preparation time: 10 minutes
Cooking time: 0 minutes
Servings: 2
Ingredients:

- 1 packet raspberry jello (sugar-free)
- 1 tsp gelatin powder
- ½ cup of boiling water
- ½ cup heavy cream

Directions:

1. Mix Jello and gelatin in boiling water in a medium bowl.
2. Stir in cream slowly and mix it for 1 minute.
3. Divide this mixture into candy molds.
4. Refrigerate them for 30 minutes.

Nutrition: Calories: 197- Fat: 19.2g - Cholesterol: 11mg - Sodium: 78 mg

229.   Cauliflower Tartar Bread

Preparation Time: 10 minutes
Cooking Time: 35 minutes
Servings: 4
Ingredients:

- 1 cup cauliflower rice
- 3 large eggs, yolks and egg whites separated
- ¼ tsp cream of tartar
- 1 ¼ cup coconut flour
- 1 ½ tbsp gluten-free baking powder
- 1 tsp sea salt
- Butter
- Cloves garlic, minced
- 1 tbsp fresh rosemary, chopped
- 1 tbsp fresh parsley, chopped

Directions:

1. Preheat your oven to 350°F. Layer a 9x5-inch pan with wax paper.
2. Place the cauliflower rice in a suitable bowl and then cover it with plastic wrap.
3. Heat it for 4 minutes in the microwave. Heat more if the cauliflower isn't soft enough.
4. Place the cauliflower rice in a kitchen towel and squeeze it to drain excess water.
5. Transfer drained cauliflower rice to a food processor.
6. Add coconut flour, sea salt, baking powder, butter, egg yolks, and garlic. Blend until crumbly.
7. Beat egg whites with cream of tartar in a bowl until foamy.
8. Add egg white mixture to the cauliflower mixture and stir well with a spatula.
9. Fold in rosemary and parsley.
10. Spread this batter in the prepared baking pan evenly.
11. Bake it for 35 minutes until golden then allow it to cool.

Nutrition: Calories: 104 - Fat: 8.9g - Carbs: 4.7g. Cholesterol: 57mg - Sodium: 340 mg.

230. Marinated Eggs

Preparation time: 2 hours and 10 minutes
Cooking time: 7 minutes
Servings: 4
Ingredients:

- Eggs
- 1 and ¼ cups water
- ¼ cup unsweetened rice vinegar
- 2 tablespoons coconut aminos
- Salt and black pepper to the taste
- 2 garlic cloves, minced
- 1 teaspoon stevia
- 4oz. cream cheese
- 1 tablespoon chives, chopped

Directions:

1. Put the eggs in a pot, add water to cover, bring to a boil over medium heat, cover and cook for 7 minutes.
2. Rinse eggs with cold water and leave them aside to cool down.
3. In a bowl, mix 1 cup water with coconut aminos, vinegar, stevia and garlic and whisk well.
4. Put the eggs in this mix, cover with a kitchen towel and leave them aside for 2 hours rotating from time to time.
5. Peel eggs, cut in halves and put egg yolks in a bowl.
6. Add ¼ cup water, cream cheese, salt, pepper and chives and stir well.
7. Stuff egg whites with this mix and serve them.

Nutrition: Calories: 289 - Protein: 15.9g - Fat: 22.6g - Carbs: 4.5g - Sodium: 288mg.

231. Pizza Balls

Preparation time: 8 minutes
Cooking time: 0
Servings: 6
Ingredients:

- 1cup fresh mozzarella
- 1cup cream cheese
- 1 tbsp olive oil
- 1 tsp tomato paste
- Large kalamata olives, pitted
- Fresh basil leaves

Directions:

1. In a food processor, mix all ingredients except basil until they form a smooth cream, about 30 seconds.
2. Form mixture into 6 balls.
3. Place 1 basil leaf on top and bottom of each ball and secure with a toothpick.
4. Serve or refrigerate up to 3 days.

Nutrition: Calories: 82 - Carbs: 0g - Fat: 8g - Protein: 3g.

232. Buttery Skillet Flatbread

Preparation Time: 10 minutes
Cooking Time: 10 minutes
Servings: 4
Ingredients:

- 1 cup almond flour
- 1 tbsp coconut flour
- 1 tsp xanthan gum
- ½ tsp baking powder
- ½ tsp salt
- 1 whole egg + 1 egg white
- 1 tbsp water (if needed)
- 1 tbsp oil, for frying
- 1 tbsp melted butter, for brushing

Directions:

1. Mix xanthan gum with flours, salt, and baking powder in a suitable bowl.
2. Beat egg and egg white in a separate bowl then stir in the flour mixture.
3. Mix well until smooth. Add a tablespoon of water if the dough is too thick.
4. Place a large skillet over medium heat and heat oil.

Nutrition: Calories: 272 - Fat: 18g - Cholesterol: 6.1mg.

233. Tasty Onion and Cauliflower Dip

Preparation time: 20 minutes
Cooking time: 30 minutes
Servings: 4
Ingredients:

- 1 and ½ cups chicken stock
- 1 cauliflower head, florets separated
- ¼ cup mayonnaise
- ½ cup yellow onion, chopped
- ¾ cup cream cheese
- ½ teaspoon chilli powder
- ½ teaspoon cumin, ground
- ½ teaspoon garlic powder
- Salt and black pepper to the taste

Directions:

1. Put the stock in a pot, add cauliflower and onion, heat up over medium heat and cook for 30 minutes.
2. Add chilli powder, salt, pepper, cumin and garlic powder and stir.
3. Also add cream cheese and stir a bit until it melts.
4. Blend using an immersion blender and mix with the mayo.
5. Transfer to a bowl and keep in the fridge for 2 hours before you serve it.

Nutrition: Calories: 40 - Protein: 1.2g - Fat: 3.3g Carbs: 1.7g - Sodium: 72mg.

234. Taco Flavored Cheddar Crisps

Preparation Time: 20 minutes
Cooking Time: 15 minutes
Servings: 6
Ingredients:

- ¾ cup sharp cheddar cheese, finely shredded
- ¼ cup parmesan cheese, finely shredded
- ¼ tbsp chilli powder
- ¼ tbsp ground cumin

Directions:

1. Preheat the oven to 400°F.
2. Line cookie sheet with parchment paper.
3. In a bowl, toss all ingredients together until well mixed.
4. Make 12 piles of cheese parchment paper.

5. Press down the cheese into a thin layer of cheese.
6. Bake for 5 minutes until cheese if bubby.
7. Allow to cool on parchment paper.
8. When completely cool, peel the paper away from the crisps.
9. These are a good intermittent substitute for chips. They are cheesy and crisp.

Nutrition: Calories: 13 - Protein: 1.4g -Fat: 0.2g Carbs: 1.4g - Sodium: 42mg.

235. Almond Garlic Crackers

Preparation time: 10 minutes
Cooking time: 15 minutes
Servings: 4
Ingredients:

- ½ cup almond flour
- ½ cup ground flaxseed
- 1/3 cup shredded Parmesan cheese
- 1 tsp. garlic powder
- ½ tsp. salt
- Water as needed

Directions:

1. Line a baking sheet with parchment paper and preheat the oven to 400°F.
2. In a bowl, mix salt, Parmesan cheese, garlic powder, water, ground flaxseed, and almond meal. Set aside for 3 to 5 minutes.
3. Put dough on the baking sheet and cover with plastic wrap. Flatten the dough with a rolling pin.
4. Remove the plastic wrap and score the dough with a knife to make dents.
5. Bake in the oven for 15 minutes.
6. Remove, cool, and break into individual crackers.

Nutrition: Calories: 96 - Fat: 14g - Carbs: 4g - Protein: 4g -Sodium: 446mg.

236.   Parmesan Crackers

Preparation time: 10 minutes
Cooking time: 5 minutes
Servings: 8
Ingredients:
- 1 tsp. butter
- 8oz. full-fat parmesan shredded

Directions:
1. Preheat the oven to 400°F.
2. Line a baking sheet with parchment paper and lightly grease the paper with the butter.
3. Spoon the parmesan cheese onto the baking sheet in mounds, spread evenly apart.
4. Spread out the mounds with the back of a spoon until they are flat.
5. Bake about 5 minutes, or until the center are still pale, and edges are browned.
6. Remove, cool, and serve.

Nutrition: Calories: 133 - Fat: 11g - Carbs: 1g - Protein: 11g - Sodium: 483mg.

237.   Deviled Eggs

Preparation time: 15 minutes
Cooking time: 10 minutes
Servings: 12
Ingredients:
- 6 Large eggs hardboiled, peeled, and halved lengthwise
- ¼ cup creamy mayonnaise
- ¼ avocado, chopped
- ¼ cup swiss cheese, shredded
- ½ tsp. dijon mustard
- Ground black pepper
- 6 bacon slices cooked and chopped

Directions
1. Remove the yolks and place them in a bowl. Place the whites on a plate, hollow side up.
2. Mash the yolks with a fork and add Dijon mustard, cheese, avocado, and mayonnaise. Mix well and season yolk mixture with the black pepper.

3. Spoon the yolk mixture back into the egg white hollows and top each egg half with the chopped bacon.
4. Serve.

Nutrition: Calories: 85 - Fat: 7g - Carbs: 2g - Protein: 6g - Sodium: 108mg.

238.   Intermittent Seed Crispy Crackers

Preparation Time: 60 minutes
Cooking Time: 55 minutes
Servings: 10
Ingredients:
- 1/3 cup almond flour
- 1/3 cup sunflower seed kernels
- 1/3 cup pumpkin seed kernels
- 1/3 cup flaxseed
- 1/3 cup chia seeds
- 1 tbsp ground psyllium husk powder
- 1 tsp salt
- ¼ cup melted coconut oil
- 1 cup boiling water

Directions:
1. Preheat the oven to 300°F:
2. Stir all dry ingredients together in a medium-sized bowl until thoroughly mixed.
3. Add coconut oil and boiling water to dry ingredients and stir until all ingredients are mixed well.
4. On a flat surface, roll the dough between two pieces of parchment paper until approximately ⅛ inch thick.
5. Slide the dough, still between parchment paper onto a baking sheet.
6. Remove the top layer of parchment paper and place dough on a baking sheet into the oven.
7. Bake 40 minutes until golden brown.
8. Score the top of the dough into cracker sized pieces.
9. Leave in the oven to cool down.
10. When the big cracker is cool, break into pieces.
11. These crackers can be stored in an airtight container after they are completely cool.

Nutrition: Calories: 61 - Carbs: 1g - Protein: 0.2g Fat: 0.6g - Sodium: 90mg.

239.   Bacon Ranch Fat Bombs

Preparation time: 15 minutes
Cooking time: 15 minutes
Servings: 4
Ingredients:
- 2oz. full-fat cream cheese, softened
- 1 tbsp ranch dressing dry mix
- 4 slices bacon

Directions:
1. Preheat the oven to 375°F.
2. Cook the bacon strips on a baking tray for 15 minutes. Let cool, then crumble.
3. In a bowl, add cream cheese and sprinkle with ranch dressing dry mix. Stir in the bacon. Mix thoroughly.
4. Form a ball out of 1 tbsp of the mixture. Repeat to form 3 more bombs. Refrigerate for 2 hours. Serve.

Nutrition: Calories: 419 - Carbs: 2.7g - Fat: 39g - Protein: 11.4g.

240.   Spicy Bacon and Avocado Balls

Preparation time: 45 minutes
Cooking time: 8 minutes
Servings: 6
Ingredients:
- 4 slices bacon
- 1 medium avocado
- 1 tbsp coconut oil
- 1 tbsp bacon fat
- 1 tbsp green onions, finely chopped
- 1 tbsp cilantro, finely chopped
- 1 small jalapeño pepper, seeded, finely chopped
- ¼ tsp sea salt

Directions:
1. Over medium heat, cook bacon until golden, about 4 minutes each side.
2. Drain bacon on a paper towel. Save bacon fat for later.
3. Once bacon is cool, chop 2 slices into crumbles.
4. Cut remaining 2 slices into 3 pieces each.
5. Smash avocado with a fork in a small bowl.

6. Add coconut oil and cooled bacon fat to avocado.
7. Add onion, cilantro, jalapeño, salt, and bacon crumbles. Blend well.
8. Refrigerate for 30 minutes.
9. Form mixture into 6 balls.
10. Place remaining 6 bacon pieces on a plate, then top each with an avocado ball.
11. Serve or refrigerate up to 3 days.

Nutrition: Calories: 181 - Carbs: 1g - Fat: 18g - Protein: 3g.

241.   Bacon, Artichoke & Onion Fat Bombs

Preparation time: 15 minutes
Cooking time: 8 minutes
Servings: 4
Ingredients:
- 4 bacon slices
- Ghee
- ½ large onion, peeled, diced
- 1 garlic clove, minced
- ⅓ cup canned artichoke hearts, sliced
- ¼ cup sour cream
- ¼ cup mayonnaise
- 1 tbsp lemon juice
- ¼ cup Swiss cheese, grated
- Salt, pepper to taste
- Avocado halves, pitted

Directions:
1. In a hot skillet, fry the bacon for 5 minutes. Let cool, then crumble.
2. Cook the onion and garlic using ghee for 3 minutes.
3. Combine the onion and garlic with the bacon and the remaining ingredients. Mix well. Season with salt and pepper. Refrigerate 30 minutes. Fill the avocado halves with the mixture and serve.

Nutrition: Calories: 408 - Carbs: 4g - Fat: 39.6g - Protein: 6.6g.

242. Brie Cheese Fat Bombs

Preparation time: 15 minutes
Cooking time: 3 minutes
Servings: 6
Ingredients:

- 8oz. full-fat cream cheese
- ¼ cup unsalted butter
- ½ cup Brie cheese, chopped
- 1 tbsp ghee
- 1 white onion, diced
- 1 garlic clove, minced
- ½ tsp paprika
- Salt, pepper to taste
- Lettuce leaves

Directions:

1. In a food processor, mix the cream cheese and butter. Transfer to a bowl. Mix in the Brie.
2. In a pan, add onion and garlic and cook 3 minutes over medium heat with ghee. Let cool. Once cooled, combine with the cheese and butter mixture.
3. Season with the spices and mix. Refrigerate 30 minutes.
4. Make 6 fat bombs out of the mixture. Serve on lettuce leaves.

Nutrition: Calories: 158 - Carbs: 1.4g - Fat: 16.2g Protein: 3.3g.

243. Salted Caramel and Brie Balls

Preparation time: 5 minutes
Cooking time: 5 minutes
Servings: 6
Ingredients:

- 9oz. brie, roughly chopped
- 1oz. salted macadamia nuts
- ½ tsp caramel flavor
- 1 tbsp butter
- 1 large apple, chopped

Directions:

1. In a food processor, mix all ingredients until a coarse mix forms, about 30 seconds.
2. Form mixture into 6 balls.

3. In a saucepan, melt the butter, then add the chopped apples. Cook until apples for about 5 minutes.
4. Spoon the apples over the brie balls. Serve or refrigerate up to 3 days.

Nutrition: Calories: 130 - Carbs: 0g - Fat: 12g - Protein: 5g.

244. Parmesan Vegetable Crips

Preparation Time: 5 minutes
Cooking Time: 10 minutes
Servings: 4
Ingredients:

- ¾ cup shredded zucchini
- ¼ cup shredded carrots
- 2 cups shredded Parmesan cheese
- 1 tbsp. olive oil
- ¼ tsp. black pepper

Directions:

1. Set the oven to 375°F. Arrange a cookie tray with parchment paper.
2. Wrap shredded vegetables in a paper towel and remove excess moisture.
3. Mix all ingredients in a bowl and mix well.
4. Put tablespoon-sized mounds onto the prepared cookie sheet.
5. Bake for 7 to 10 minutes until lightly browned.
6. Let it cool for at least 2 to 3 minutes and serve.

Nutrition: Calories: 206 - Fat: 14g - Carbs: 3.6g - Protein: 15.8g.

245. Nori Snack Rolls

Preparation Time: 5 minutes
Cooking Time: 10 minutes
Servings: 4
Ingredients:

- 2 tablespoons almond, cashew, peanut, or another nut butter
- 2 tablespoons tamari, or soy sauce
- Standard nori sheets
- 1 mushroom, sliced
- 1 tablespoon pickled ginger
- ½ cup grated carrots

Directions:

1. Set the oven to 350°F.
2. Combine together the nut butter and tamari until smooth and very thick. Layout a nori sheet, rough side up, the long way.
3. Spread a thin line of the tamari mixture on the far end of the nori sheet, from side to side. Lay the mushroom slices, ginger, and carrots in a line at the other end (the end closest to you).
4. Fold the vegetables inside the nori, rolling toward the tahini mixture, which will seal the roll. Repeat to make 4 rolls.
5. Bring on a baking sheet, then bake for 8 to 10 minutes, or the rolls are slightly browned and crispy at the ends. Let the rolls cool for a few minutes, then slice each roll into 3 smaller pieces.

Nutrition: Calories: 79 - Fat: 5g - Carbs: 6g - Fibre: 2g - Protein: 4g.

246. Risotto Bites

Preparation Time: 15 minutes
Cooking Time: 20 minutes
Servings: 12
Ingredients:

- ½ cup breadcrumbs
- 1 tsp. paprika
- 1 tsp. chipotle powder or ground cayenne pepper
- 1½ cups cold Green Pea Risotto
- Nonstick cooking spray

Directions:

1. Set the oven to 425°F.
2. Line a baking sheet using parchment paper.
3. On a large plate, put and combine the panko, paprika, and chipotle powder. Set aside.
4. Make the 2 tablespoons of the risotto into a ball.
5. Roll in the breadcrumbs, then put on the prepared baking sheet. Repeat to make a total of 12 balls.
6. Spray the tops of the risotto bites with nonstick cooking spray then bake for at least 15 to 20 minutes until it starts to brown. Cool it before storing it in a large airtight container in a single layer.

Nutrition: Calories: 100 - Fat: 2g - Protein: 6g - Carbs: 17g - Fibre: 5g - Sugar: 2g - Sodium: 165mg.

247. Intermittent Popcorn Cheese Puffs

Preparation Time: 10 minutes
Cooking Time: 8 minutes (Resting Time 3 days)
Servings: 5
Ingredients:

- 8oz. cheddar cheese sliced

Directions:

1. Cut the cheddar into small ¼-inch squares and place on a baking sheet.
2. Cover the baking sheet with parchment paper.
3. Let the cheddar dry for 3 days.
4. Preheat the oven to 350°F. and reheat the cheddar for 5-8 minutes until it swells and turns golden on the edges.
5. Leave to cool for 10 minutes before serving.

Nutrition: Calories: 183 - Fat: 15g - Carbs: 2g - Protein: 10g.

248. Black Sesame Wonton Chips

Preparation Time: 5 minutes
Cooking Time: 5 minutes
Servings: 3
Ingredients:

- 6 vegan wonton wrappers
- 1 ½ teaspoons toasted sesame oil
- 1/3 cup black sesame seeds
- Salt

Directions:

1. Preheat the oven to 425°F. Lightly grease with oil a baking sheet and set aside. Cut the wonton wrappers in half crosswise, brush them with sesame oil, and arrange them in a single layer on the prepared baking sheet.
2. Sprinkle wonton wrappers with the sesame seeds and salt to taste, and bake until crisp and golden brown, 5 to 7 minutes. Cool completely before serving.

Nutrition: Calories: 62 - Protein: 3g - Fat: 3g - Carbs: 8g.

249. Curried Tofu "Egg Salad" Pitas

Preparation Time: 15 minutes
Cooking Time: 0 minutes
Servings: 4
Ingredients:

- 1lb. extra-firm tofu, drained and patted dry
- ½ cup vegan mayonnaise, homemade or store-bought
- ¼ cup chopped mango chutney, homemade or store-bought
- 2 teaspoons Dijon mustard
- 1 tablespoon hot or mild curry powder
- 1 teaspoon salt
- 1/8 teaspoon ground cayenne
- ¾ cup shredded carrots
- Celery ribs, minced
- ¼ cup minced red onion
- Small Boston or other soft lettuce leaves
- 7-inch whole-wheat pita bread, halved

Directions:

1. Crumble the tofu then put it in a large bowl. Add the mayonnaise, chutney, mustard, curry powder, salt, and cayenne, and stir well until thoroughly mixed.
2. Add the carrots, celery, and onion and stir to combine. Refrigerate for 30 minutes to allow the flavors to blend.
3. Tuck a lettuce leaf inside each pita pocket, spoon some tofu mixture on top of the lettuce and serve.

Nutrition: Calories: 533 - Protein: 26.1g - Fat: 29.4g - Carbs: 50.6g.

250. Tamari Toasted Almonds

Preparation Time: 2 minutes
Cooking Time: 8 minutes
Servings: 4
Ingredients:

- ½ cup raw almonds, or sunflower seeds
- 2 tablespoons tamari, or soy sauce
- 1 teaspoon toasted sesame oil

Directions:

1. Heat a dry skillet to medium-high heat, then add the almonds, stirring very frequently to keep them from burning. Once the almonds are toasted, 7 to 8 minutes for almonds, or 3 to 4 minutes for sunflower seeds, pour the tamari and sesame oil into the hot skillet and stir to coat.
2. You can turn off the heat, and as the almonds cool, the tamari mixture will stick to and dry on the nuts.

Nutrition: Calories: 89 - Fat: 8g - Carbs: 3g - Fibre: 2g - Protein: 4g.

Chapter 15. Smoothies and Drinks

251. Vanilla Intermittent Smoothie

Preparation Time: 11 minutes
Cooking Time: 0 minutes
Servings: 2
Ingredients:
- 13.5oz. can coconut milk
- 1 cup heavy cream
- ¼ cup sweetener or to taste
- 1 tsp vanilla extract
- 2 cups ice cubes

Directions:
1. Put all together the ingredients in a blender and blend until pureed.

Nutrition: Calories: 379 - Fat: 38g - Carbs: 4g - Protein: 3g.

252. Cinnamon Raspberry Smoothie

Preparation Time: 11 minutes
Cooking Time: 0 minutes
Servings: 1
Ingredients:
- ½ cup of unsweetened almond milk
- ½ cup of frozen raspberries
- 1 cup of spinach
- 1 tbsp. of almond butter
- 1/8 tsp of cinnamon

Directions:
1. Place all the ingredients into the blender and blend until pureed.
2. Enjoy as breakfast or snacks.

Nutrition: Calories: 286 - Fat: 21g - Carbs: 19g - Protein: 10g.

253. Bulletproof Coffee

Preparation Time: 5 minutes
Cooking Time: 0 minutes
Servings: 1
Ingredients:
- 1 tbsp. MCT oil powder
- 1 tbsp. Ghee/butter
- 1 cup of hot coffee and dilute it a little with hot water

Directions:
1. Empty the hot coffee into your blender.
2. Pour in the powder and butter. Blend until frothy.
3. Enjoy in a large mug.

Nutrition: Calorie: 463 - Protein: 1g - Fat: 51g - Carbs: 0g.

254. Peanut Butter Caramel Milkshake

Preparation Time: 5 minutes
Cooking Time: 0 minutes
Servings: 1
Ingredients:
- 1 tbsp. natural peanut butter
- 1 tbsp. MCT Oil
- 0.25 tsp. xanthan gum
- 1 cup coconut milk
- Ice cubes
- 1 tbsp. sugar-free salted caramel syrup

Directions:
1. Combine each of the components in a blender.
2. Mix thoroughly and serve in a chilled mug.

Nutrition: Calorie: 365 - Protein: 8g - Fat: 35g - Carbs: 5g.

255.   Strawberry Almond Smoothie

Preparation Time: 10 minutes
Cooking Time: 0 minutes
Servings: 2
Ingredients:

- 0.25 cup Frozen unsweetened strawberries
- 1 tbsp. Whey vanilla isolate powder
- 0.5 cup Heavy cream
- 16oz. unsweetened almond milk
- Stevia (as desired)

Directions:

1. Toss or pour each of the fixings into a blender.
2. Puree until smooth.
3. Pour a small amount of water to thin the smoothie as needed.

Nutrition: Calorie: 34 - Protein: 15g - Fat: 25g - Carbs: 7g.

256.   Blueberry Coconut Chia Smoothies

Preparation Time: 11 minutes
Cooking Time: 0 minutes
Servings: 4
Ingredients:

- 1 cup frozen blueberries
- 1 cup full-fat Greek yogurt
- ½ cup coconut cream
- 1 cup unsweetened cashew or almond milk
- 1 tbsp. coconut oil
- 1 tbsp. ground chia seed
- 1 tbsp. swerve sweetener

Directions:

1. To a high-speed blender, add all the smoothie ingredients and blend until smooth and combined.
2. Serve immediately and enjoy!

Nutrition: Calories: 249 - Fat: 21.1g - Carbs: 11.3g - Protein: 6.2g.

257.   Strawberry Zucchini Chia Smoothie

Preparation Time: 11 minutes
Cooking Time: 0 minutes
Servings: 1
Ingredients:

- 1 cup of water
- ½ cup of frozen strawberries
- 1 cup of chopped zucchini, frozen or raw
- 1 tbsp. of chia seeds

Directions:

1. To a high-speed blender, add all the smoothie ingredients and blend until smooth and combined.
2. Serve immediately and enjoy!

Nutrition: Calories: 198 - Fat: 9g - Carbs: 9g - Protein: 7g.

258.   Chocolate Peanut Butter Smoothie

Preparation Time: 5 minutes
Cooking Time: 0 minutes
Servings: 3
Ingredients:

- ¼ cup peanut butter (creamy)
- 1 tbsp. cocoa powder
- 1 cup heavy cream
- 1 ½ cup unsweetened almond milk
- 1 tbsp. sweetener to taste
- 1/8 tsp sea salt (optional)

Directions:

1. To a high-speed blender, add all the smoothie ingredients and blend until smooth and combined.
2. Serve immediately and enjoy!

Nutrition: Calories: 435 - Fat: 41g - Carbs: 6g - Protein: 9g.

259. Strawberry Shake

Preparation Time: 5 minutes
Cooking Time: 0 minutes
Servings: 2
Ingredients:

- ½ cup almond milk
- ½ cup coconut milk, unsweetened or heavy whipping cream
- 8oz. strawberries
- 2 tablespoons sugar- free vanilla syrup
- 2 tablespoons coconut oil
- Whipped cream or coconut cream, (optional)
- Chia seeds (optional)

Directions:

1. Put all together the ingredients in a blender, and blend until you obtain a smooth mixture.
2. Put into tall glasses and serve topped with whipped cream if using.

Nutrition: Calories 276 - Fat: 27.4g - Protein: 2.5g - Carbs: 6.4g.

260. Spinach & Avocado Smoothie

Preparation Time: 10 minutes
Cooking Time: 0 minutes
Servings: 2
Ingredients:

- ½ large avocado, peeled, pitted, and roughly chopped
- 2 cups fresh spinach
- 1 tablespoon MCT oil
- 1 teaspoon organic vanilla extract
- 6 - 8 drops liquid stevia
- 1½ cups unsweetened almond milk
- ½ cup ice cubes

Directions:

1. In a blender, put all the listed ingredients and pulse until creamy.
2. Pour the smoothie into two glasses and serve immediately.

Nutrition: Calories: 180 - Carbs: 0g - Fat: 9g - Protein: 2.4g - Cholesterol: 0mg - Sodium: 161mg - Fibre: 4.3g - Sugar: 0.6g.

261. Blueberry Yogurt Smoothie

Preparation Time: 5 minutes
Cooking Time: 0 minutes
Servings: 2
Ingredients:

- 1 cup blueberries
- 1 cup coconut milk
- Stevia (to taste)

Directions:

1. Combine all of the fixings in the blender. Mix well.
2. When creamy, pour into two chilled glasses and enjoy.

Nutrition: Calorie: 70 - Protein: 2g - Fat: 5g - Carbs: 2g.

262. Almond Smoothie

Preparation Time: 10 minutes
Cooking Time: 0 minutes
Servings: 2
Ingredients:

- ¾ cup almonds, chopped
- ½ cup heavy whipping cream
- 2 teaspoons butter, melted
- ¼ teaspoon organic vanilla extract
- 7–8 drops liquid stevia
- 1 cup unsweetened almond milk
- ¼ cup ice cubes

Directions:

1. In a blender, put all the listed ingredients and pulse until creamy.
2. Pour the smoothie into two glasses and serve immediately.

Nutrition: Calories: 365 - Carbs: 4.5g - Fat: 10.8g Fibre: 5g - Cholesterol: 51mg - Sodium: 129mg - Protein: 8.7g.

263. Strawberry Smoothie

Preparation Time: 10 minutes
Cooking Time: 0 minutes
Servings: 2
Ingredients:

- 2cups frozen strawberries
- 2 teaspoons granulated erythritol
- ½ teaspoon organic vanilla extract
- 1/3 cup heavy whipping cream
- 1¼ cups unsweetened almond milk
- ½ cup ice cubes

Directions:

1. In a blender, put all the listed ingredients and pulse until creamy.
2. Pour the smoothie into two glasses and serve immediately.

Nutrition: Calories: 115 - Carbs: 4.5g - Fat: 4.8 g Protein: 1.4g - Cholesterol: 2m - Sodium: 121mg Fibre: 1.8g - Sugar: 2.9g.

264. Raspberry Smoothie

Preparation Time: 10 minutes
Cooking Time: 0 minutes
Servings: 2
Ingredients:

- ¾ cup fresh raspberries
- 4 tablespoons heavy whipping cream
- 1/3oz. cream cheese
- 1 cup unsweetened almond milk
- ½ cup ice, crushed

Directions:

1. In a blender, put all the listed ingredients and pulse until creamy.
2. Pour the smoothie into two glasses and serve immediately.

Nutrition: Calories 138 - Carbs: 3.8g - Fat: 6.4g - Protein: 1.9g - Cholesterol: 36mg - Sodium: 115mg - Fibre: 3.5g - Sugar: 2.1g.

265. Pumpkin Smoothie

Preparation Time: 10 minutes
Cooking Time: 0 minutes
Servings: 2
Ingredients:

- ½ cup homemade pumpkin puree
- 6oz. cream cheese, softened
- ¼ cup heavy cream
- ½ teaspoon pumpkin pie spice
- ¼ teaspoon ground cinnamon
- 6-8 drops liquid stevia
- 2 tsp organic vanilla extract
- 1 cup unsweetened almond milk
- ¼ cup ice cubes

Directions:

1. In a blender, put all the listed ingredients and pulse until creamy.
2. Pour the smoothie into two glasses and serve immediately.

Nutrition: Calories: 296 - Carbs: 5.4g - Fat: 16.1g Protein: 5.6g - Cholesterol: 83mg - Sodium: 266mg - Fibre: 2.6g - Sugar: 2.4g.

266. Mocha Smoothie

Preparation Time: 10 minutes
Cooking Time: 0 minutes
Servings: 2
Ingredients:

- 1 ½ cup chocolate almond milk
- 2 bananas
- 2 tablespoon ground espresso powder
- 1/2 teaspoon ground cinnamon
- 8oz. plain greek yogurt
- 2 scoop vanilla protein powder
- 3 cup ice cubes

Directions:

1. Add all the ingredients to a blender. Blend until smooth and serve!

Nutrition: Calories: 360 - Carbs: 57g - Fat: 3g - Cholesterol: 20mg - Sodium: 240mg - Fibre: 4g - Sugar: 40g - Protein: 30g.

267.   Creamy Spinach Smoothie

Preparation Time: 10 minutes
Cooking Time: 0 minutes
Servings: 2
Ingredients:

- 2 cups fresh baby spinach
- 1 tablespoon almond butter
- 1 tablespoon chia seeds
- 1/8 teaspoon ground cinnamon
- Pinch of ground cloves
- ½ cup heavy cream
- 1 cup unsweetened almond milk
- ½ cup ice cubes

Directions:

1. In a blender, put all the listed Ingredients: and pulse until creamy.
2. Pour the smoothie into two glasses and serve immediately.

Nutrition: Calories: 195 - Carbs: 2.8g - Fat: 7.5g Protein: 4.5g - Cholesterol: 41mg - Sodium: 126mg - Fibre: 3.3g - Sugar: 0.5g.

268.   Matcha Smoothie

Preparation Time: 10 minutes
Cooking Time: 0 minutes
Servings: 2
Ingredients:

- 2 tablespoons chia seeds
- 2 teaspoons matcha green tea powder
- ½ teaspoon fresh lemon juice
- ½ teaspoon xanthan gum
- 6 - 8 drops liquid stevia
- 2 tablespoons plain Greek yogurt
- 1½ cups unsweetened almond milk
- ¼ cup ice cubes

Directions:

1. In a blender, put all the listed ingredients and pulse until creamy.
2. Pour the smoothie into two glasses and serve immediately.

Nutrition: Calories: 85 - Carbs: 3.5g - Fat: 0.8g - Protein: 4g - Cholesterol: 2mg - Sodium: 174mg Fibre: 4.1g - Sugar: 2.2g.

269.   Coconut Milk Strawberry Smoothie

Preparation Time: 2 minutes
Cooking Time: 0 minutes
Servings: 2
Ingredients:

- 1 cup strawberries frozen
- 1 cup unsweetened coconut milk
- 1 tbsp. smooth almond butter
- Stevia (optional)

Directions:

1. Place all together the ingredients into the food processor and blend until pureed.

Nutrition: Calories: 397 - Fat: 37g - Carbs: 15g - Protein: 6g.

Chapter 16. Desserts

270. Cookie Ice Cream

Preparation time: 5 minutes
Cooking time: 2 hours
Servings: 2
Ingredients:
Cookie Crumbs:
- ¾ cup almond flour
- ¼ cup cocoa powder
- ¼ tsp baking soda
- ¼ cup erythritol
- ½ tsp vanilla extract
- ½ tbsp coconut oil, softened
- 1 large egg, room temperature
- Pinch of salt

Ice Cream:
- ½ cup whipping cream
- 1 tbsp vanilla extract
- ½ cup erythritol
- ½ cup almond milk, unsweetened

Directions:
1. Preheat your oven at 300°F and layer a 9-inch baking pan with wax paper.
2. Whisk almond flour with baking soda, cocoa powder, salt, and erythritol in a medium bowl.
3. Stir in coconut oil and vanilla extract then mix well until crumbly.
4. Whisk in egg and mix well to form the dough.
5. Spread this dough in the prepared pan and bake for 20 minutes in the preheated oven.
6. Allow the crust to cool then crush it finely into crumbles.
7. Beat cream in a large bowl with a hand mixer until it forms a stiff peak.
8. Stir in erythritol and vanilla extract then mix well until fully incorporated.
9. Pour in milk and blend well until smooth.
10. Add this mixture to an ice cream machine and churn as per the machine's instructions.
11. Add cookie crumbles to the ice cream in the machine and churn again.
12. Place the ice cream in a sealable container and freeze for 2 hours.
13. Scoop out the ice cream and serve.
14. Enjoy.

Nutrition: Calories: 214 - Fat 5.8g - Carbs: 6g - Cholesterol 15mg - Protein: 6.5g - Fibre: 2.1g - Sodium: 123mg - Sugar: 1.9g.

271. Intermittent Vanilla Ice Cream

Preparation time: 8 hours and 5 minutes
Cooking time: 0
Servings: 8
Ingredients:
- 2 (15oz.) cans coconut milk
- 1 cup heavy cream
- ¼ cup Swerve confectioner's sweetener
- 1 tsp pure vanilla extract
- Pinch kosher salt

Directions:
1. Refrigerate coconut milk for 3 hours or overnight and remove the cream from the top while leaving the liquid in the can. Place the cream in a bowl.
2. Beat the coconut cream using a hand mixer until it forms peaks.
3. Stir in vanilla, sweeteners, and whipped cream then beat well until fluffy.
4. Freeze this mixture for 5 hours.
5. Enjoy.

Nutrition: Calories: 255 - Fat: 11.7g - Carbs: 2.5g Sugar: 12.5g - Protein: 7.9g - Cholesterol: 135mg Sodium: 112mg - Fibre: 1g.

272.   Flourless Chocolate Torte

Preparation time: 10 minutes
Cooking time: 20 minutes
Servings: 6
Ingredients:

- Cooking oil spray, for greasing
- 1½ cups plus 2 tablespoons water, divided
- 7oz. sugar-free dark chocolate
- ¼ cup low-Carbs sugar substitute, such as Swerve
- ½lb. unsalted butter, room temperature
- 4 eggs
- Pinch salt

Directions:

1. Grease an 8-by-2-inch cake pan with the cooking oil spray.
2. In a saucepan over medium-low heat, add 2 tablespoons of water, the chocolate, and sweetener. Heat, stirring frequently, until smooth and well-combined. Add the butter and stir gently until melted. Remove the pan from the heat.
3. In a large bowl, whisk the eggs until smooth. Slowly whisk the eggs and salt into the chocolate mixture, being careful to incorporate slowly so the warm chocolate doesn't scramble the eggs. Pour the mixture into the prepared cake pan.
4. Place the remaining 1½ cups of water in the pot. Place the reversible rack in the pot, making sure it is in the steaming position. Carefully place the cake pan on the rack. Assemble the pressure lid, making sure the pressure release valve is in the seal position.
5. Select pressure and set to high. Set time to 6 minutes. Select start/stop to begin.
6. When pressure cooking is complete, quick release the pressure by moving the pressure release valve to the vent position. Carefully remove the lid when the unit has finished releasing pressure.
7. Carefully remove the pan using an oven mitt. Let cool on the counter before

refrigerating for at least 4 hours. I like to pop it in the freezer before serving.

Nutrition: Calories: 705 - Fat: 65g - Fibre: 10g - Carbs: 3g - Protein: 14g.

273.   Pumpkin Pie Pudding

Preparation time: 5 minutes
Cooking time: 15 minutes
Servings: 6
Ingredients:

- Unsalted butter, room temperature, or cooking oil spray, for greasing
- 15oz. pumpkin purée
- 1 teaspoon liquid stevia
- 1 tablespoon cinnamon
- 1 teaspoon ground nutmeg
- 1 teaspoon ground ginger
- 1 teaspoon ground allspice
- 2 eggs yolks
- ¾ cup heavy (whipping) cream
- 1 cup water

Directions:

1. Grease 6 ramekins with the butter.
2. In a large bowl, combine the pumpkin purée, stevia, cinnamon, nutmeg, ginger, allspice, egg yolks, and cream and mix until smooth. Pour into the prepared ramekins.
3. Place the reversible rack in the pot, making sure it is in the steaming position. Place the water in the pot and place the ramekins on rack. Fit the bonnet, making sure the pressure release valve is in the sealed position.
4. Select pressure and set to high. Set time to 7 minutes. Select start/stop to begin.
5. When cooking is complete, release the pressure by moving the release valve to the vent position. Remove the cover
6. when the unit has finished releasing pressure.
7. Remove the ramekins and let rest/cool for at least 10 minutes before serving.

Nutrition: Calories: 170 - Fat: 14g - Fibre: 3g - Carbs: 5g - Protein: 3g.

274.   Orange Custard Cups

Preparation time: 4 hours and 20 minutes
Cooking time: 5 minutes
Servings: 5
Ingredients:

- 3 cups coconut milk, full fat
- 2 eggs
- ¼ cup fresh orange juice
- 1 medium orange, zested
- 3 scoops intermittent collagen, grass-fed
- 2 teaspoons vanilla extract, unsweetened
- 1/8 teaspoon erythritol sweetener
- Salt
- 1 ½ scoop gelatin, pastured
- 1 cup water

Directions:

1. Place all the ingredients in a food processor except for the gelatin and water, pulse until smooth, then add gelatin and blend until smooth.
2. Divide the custard evenly between five half-pint jars and cover with their lid.
3. Switch on the instant pot, pour in water, insert trivet stand, place jars on it and shut the instant pot with its lid in the sealed position.
4. Press the 'manual' button, press '+/-' to the set the cooking time to 5 minutes and cook at high-pressure setting; when the pressure builds in the pot, the cooking timer will start.
5. When the instant pot buzzes, press the 'keep warm' button, do a quick pressure release and open the lid.
6. Carefully remove the jars, let them cool at room temperature for 15 minutes or more until they can be comfortably picked up.
7. Then transfer the custard jars into the refrigerator for a minimum of 4 hours and cool completely.
8. When ready to serve, shake the jars a few times to mix all the ingredients and then serve.

Nutrition: Calories: 250 - Fat: 24g - Protein: 5g - Carbs: 2g - Fibre: 3g.

275.   Mocha Mousse

Preparation time: 2 hours and 35 minutes
Cooking time: 0
Servings: 4
Ingredients:
For the Cream Cheese:

- 8oz. cream cheese, softened and full fat
- 3 tablespoons sour cream, full fat
- 2 tablespoons butter, softened
- 1 ½ teaspoons vanilla extract, unsweetened
- 1/3 cup erythritol
- ¼ cup cocoa powder, unsweetened
- 3 teaspoons instant coffee powder

For the Whipped Cream:

- 2/3 cup heavy whipping cream, full fat
- 1 ½ teaspoon erythritol
- ½ teaspoon vanilla extract, unsweetened

Directions:

1. Prepare cream cheese mixture: For this, place cream cheese in a bowl, add sour cream and butter then beat until smooth.
2. Now add erythritol, cocoa powder, coffee, and vanilla and blend until incorporated, set aside until required.
3. Prepare whipping cream: For this, place whipping cream in a bowl and beat until soft peaks form.
4. Beat in vanilla and erythritol until stiff peaks form, then add 1/3 of the mixture into cream cheese mixture and fold until just mixed.
5. Then add remaining whipping cream mixture and fold until evenly incorporated.
6. Spoon the mousse into a freezer-proof bowl and place in the refrigerator for 2 ½ hours until set.
7. Serve straight away.

Nutrition: Calories: 422 - Fat: 42g - Protein: 6g - Carbs: 6.5g - Fibre: 2g.

276. Strawberry Rhubarb Custard

Preparation time: 4 hours and 5 minutes
Cooking time: 5 minutes
Servings: 5
Ingredients:

- 27oz. coconut milk, full fat
- 2 eggs
- ¾ cup strawberries, fresh
- ½ cup rhubarb, chopped
- ¼ cup collagen, grass-fed
- 1 teaspoon vanilla extract, unsweetened
- 1/16 teaspoon stevia, liquid
- Salt
- 1 ½ tablespoons gelatin, grass-fed
- 1 cup water

Directions:

1. Place all the ingredients in a food processor except for the gelatin and water, pulse until smooth, then add gelatin and blend until smooth.
2. Divide the custard evenly between five half-pint jars and cover with their lid.
3. Switch on the instant pot, pour in water, insert trivet stand, place jars on it and shut the instant pot with its lid the in the sealed position.
4. Press the 'manual' button, press '+/-' to set the cooking time to 5 minutes and cook at high-pressure setting; when the pressure builds in the pot, the cooking timer will start.
5. When the instant pot buzzes, press the 'keep warm' button, do a quick pressure release and open the lid.
6. Carefully remove the jars, let them cool at room temperature for 15 minutes or more until they can be comfortably picked up.
7. Then transfer the custard jars into the refrigerator for a minimum of 4 hours and cool completely.
8. When ready to serve, shake the jars a few times to mix all the ingredients and then serve.

Nutrition: Calories: 262 - Fat: 24g Carbs: 3g Protein: 5g - Fibre: 3g.

277. Chocolate Avocado Ice Cream

Preparation time: 12 hours and 10 minutes
Cooking time: 0
Servings: 6
Ingredients:

- 2 large organic avocados, pitted
- ½ cup erythritol, powdered
- ½ cup cocoa powder, organic and unsweetened
- 25 drops of liquid stevia
- 2 teaspoons vanilla extract, unsweetened
- 1 cup coconut milk, full-fat and unsweetened
- ½ cup heavy whipping cream, full fat
- 6 squares of chocolate, unsweetened and chopped

Directions:

1. Scoop out the flesh from each avocado, place it in a bowl and add vanilla, milk, and cream and blend using an immersion blender until smooth and creamy.
2. Add remaining ingredients except for chocolate and mix until well combined and smooth.
3. Fold in chopped chocolate and let the mixture chill in the refrigerator for 8 to 12 hours or until cooled.
4. When ready to serve, let ice cream stand for 30 minutes at room temperature, then process it using an ice cream machine as per manufacturer instruction.
5. Serve immediately.

Nutrition: Calories: 217 - Fat: 19.4g - Carbs: 3.7g Protein: 3.8g - Fibre: 7.4g.

278. Key Lime Curd

Preparation time: 4 hours and 30 minutes
Cooking time: 10 minutes
Servings: 3
Ingredients:
- 3oz. butter, unsalted
- 1 cup erythritol sweetener
- 2 eggs
- 2 eggs yolks
- 2/3 cup key lime juice
- 2 teaspoons key lime zest
- 1 ½ cups water

Directions:
1. Place butter in a food processor, add sugar, blend for 2 minutes, then add eggs and yolks and continue blending for 1 minute.
2. Add lime juice, blend until combined and a smooth curd comes together and then pour the mixture evenly into three half-pint mason jars.
3. Switch on the instant pot, pour in water, insert a trivet stand, place mason jars on it and shut the instant pot with its lid the in the sealed position.
4. Press the 'manual' button, press '+/-' to set the cooking time to 10 minutes and cook at high-pressure setting; when the pressure builds in the pot, the cooking timer will start.
5. When the instant pot buzzes, press the 'keep warm' button, release pressure naturally for 10 minutes, then do a quick pressure release and open the lid.
6. Remove jars from the instant pot, open them, add lime zest, stir until combined and then close the jars with their lids again.
7. Let the jars cool at room temperature for 20 minutes, then place them in the refrigerator for 4 hours or more until chilled and curd gets thickened.
8. Serve straight away.

Nutrition: Calories: 78 - Fat: 4.5g - Protein: 7g - Carbs: 1g - Fibre:1g.

279. Butter Pecan Ice Cream

Preparation time: 5 minutes
Cooking time: 5 minutes
Servings: 3
Ingredients:
- ½ cup unsweetened coconut milk
- ¼ cup heavy whipping cream
- 1 tbsp butter
- ¼ cup crushed pecans
- 25 drops liquid stevia
- ¼ tsp xanthan gum

Directions:
1. Place a pan over medium-low heat and melt butter in it until it turns brown.
2. Mix this butter with chopped pecans, heavy cream, and stevia in a bowl.
3. Stir in coconut milk then xanthan gum and mix well until fluffy.
4. Add this mixture to an ice cream machine and churn as per the machine's instructions.
5. Once done, serve.

Nutrition: Calories: 251 - Fat: 14.7g - Sugar: 0.5g Protein: 5.9g - Carbs: 4.3g - Cholesterol: 16 mg - Sodium: 142mg - Fibre: 1g.

280. Creamy Hot Chocolate

Preparation Time: 5 minutes
Cooking Time: 5 minutes
Servings: 2
Ingredients:
- 4oz. dark chocolate, chopped
- ½ cup unsweetened almond milk
- ½ cup heavy cream
- 1 tbsp. erythritol
- ½ tsp vanilla extract

Directions:
1. Combine the almond milk, erythritol, and cream in a small saucepan. Heat it (choose medium heat and cook for 1-2 minutes).
2. Add vanilla extract and chocolate. Stir continuously until the chocolate melts.
3. Pour into cups and serve.

Nutrition: Calories: 193 - Carbs: 4 g - Fat: 18g - Protein: 2g.

281. Almond Meal Cupcakes

Preparation time: 15 minutes
Cooking time: 15 minutes
Servings: 12
Ingredients:

- ½ cup almond meal
- ¼ cup butter, melted
- 8oz. cream cheese, softened
- 6 eggs
- ¾ teaspoon liquid stevia
- teaspoon vanilla extract

Special equipment:

- A 12-cup muffin pan

Directions:

1. Preheat your oven to 350°F. Line a muffin pan with 12 paper liners.
2. Thoroughly mix the almond meal with butter in a bowl, then spoon this mixture into the bottoms of each paper liner and press it into a thin crust.
3. Make the cupcakes: Whisk the cream cheese with liquid stevia, eggs, and vanilla extract in a medium bowl. Beat with an electric beater until the mixture is fluffy, creamy and smooth. Spoon this filling over the crust layer in the muffin pan.
4. Bake in the preheated oven until the cream cheese mixture is cooked from the center, for 15 to 17 minutes.
5. Leave the cupcakes to cool at room temperature. Serve immediately or refrigerate to chill for 8 hours, preferably overnight.

Nutrition: Calories:199 - Fat: 19.1g - Carbs: 2.6g Fibre: 0.5g - Protein: 4.7g.

282. Almond Cinnamon Cookies

Preparation time: 10 minutes
Cooking time: 15 minutes
Servings: 2
Ingredients:

- 1 ½ cups blanched almond flour
- ½ cup butter, softened
- 1 egg
- ½ cup swerve
- 1 teaspoon sugar-free vanilla extract
- 1 teaspoon ground cinnamon

Directions:

1. Preheat your oven to 350°F. Layer a baking sheet with parchment paper.
2. Whisk the almond flour with butter, vanilla extract, Swerve, egg, and cinnamon in a bowl. Mix well until these ingredients form a smooth dough.
3. Make the cookies: Divide the dough and roll it into 1-inch balls on a lightly floured surface. Arrange these balls on the prepared baking sheet and press each ball lightly with a fork to make a crisscross pattern.
4. Bake these cinnamon cookies in the preheated oven for 12 to 15 minutes, or until their edges turn golden.
5. Allow the cinnamon cookies to cool on the baking sheet for 5 minutes, then transfer them to a wire rack to cool completely before serving.

Nutrition: Calories: 92 - Fat: 7.4g - Carbs: 3.0g - Fibre: 0.1g - Protein: 3.4g.

283. Cream Cheese Chocolate Mousse

Preparation time: 10 minutes
Cooking time: 0
Servings: 2
Ingredients:

- 3oz. cream cheese, softened
- ½ cup heavy cream
- 1 teaspoon vanilla extract
- ¼ cup Swerve
- 2 tablespoons cocoa powder
- Pinch salt

Directions:

1. Beat the cream cheese in a large mixing bowl with an electric beater until it makes fluffy mixture.
2. Switch the beater to low speed, and add the vanilla extract, heavy cream, salt, Swerve, and cocoa powder to beat for 2 minutes until it is completely smooth.
3. Chill in the refrigerator until ready to serve.

Nutrition: Calories: 270 - Fat: 26.4g - Carbs: 6.0g - Fibre: 2.0g - Protein: 4.2g.

284. Sugar-Free Lemon Bars

Preparation Time: 15 minutes
Cooking Time: 45 minutes
Servings: 8
Ingredients:

- ½ cup butter, melted
- 1¾ cup almond flour, divided
- 1 cup powdered erythritol, divided
- Medium-size lemons
- 4 large eggs

Directions:

1. Prepare the parchment paper and baking tray. Combine butter, 1 cup of almond flour, ¼ cup of erythritol, and salt. Stir well. Place the mix on the baking sheet, press a little and put it into the oven (preheated to 350°F). Cook for about 20 minutes. Then set aside to let it cool.
2. Zest 1 lemon and juice all of the lemons in a bowl. Add the eggs, ¾ cup of erythritol, ¾ cup of almond flour, and

salt. Stir together to create the filling. Pour it on top of the cake and cook for 25 minutes. Cut into small pieces and serve with lemon slices.

Nutrition: Calories: 272 - Carbs: 4g - Fat: 26g - Protein: 8g.

285. Vanilla Almond Ice Pops

Preparation Time: 10 minutes + 4 hours chilling
Cooking Time: 15 minutes
Servings: 18
Ingredients:

- 2 cups almond milk
- 1 cup heavy (whipping) cream
- 1 vanilla bean, halved lengthwise
- 1 cup shredded unsweetened coconut

Directions:

1. Set a medium saucepan on medium heat, then put the almond milk, heavy cream, and vanilla bean.
2. Bring the liquid to a simmer and reduce the heat to low. Continue to simmer for 5 minutes.
3. Remove the saucepan from the heat and let the liquid cool.
4. Take the vanilla bean out of the liquid and use a knife to scrape the seeds out of the bean into the liquid.
5. Stir in the coconut and divide the liquid between the ice pop molds.
6. Freeze until solid, about 4 hours, and enjoy.

Nutrition: Calories: 166 - Fat: 15g - Protein: 3g - Carbs: 4g - Fibre: 2g.

286. Fatty Bombs with Cinnamon and Cardamom

Preparation Time: 10 minutes
Cooking Time: 35 minutes
Servings: 2
Ingredients:

- ½ cup unsweetened coconut, shredded
- 2.5oz unsalted butter
- ¼ tsp ground green cinnamon
- ¼ ground cardamom
- ½ tsp vanilla extract

Directions:

1. Roast the unsweetened coconut (choose medium-high heat) until it begins to turn lightly brown.
2. Combine the room-temperature butter, half of the shredded coconut, cinnamon, cardamom, and vanilla extract in a separate dish. Cool the mix in the fridge for about 5-10 minutes.
3. Form small balls and cover them with the remaining shredded coconut.
4. Cool the balls in the fridge for about 10-15 minutes.

Nutrition: Calories: 90 - Carbs: 0.4g - Fat: 10g - Protein: 0.4g.

287. Vanilla Mug Cake

Preparation time: 5 minutes
Cooking time: 5 minutes
Servings: 1
Ingredients:

- 1 tablespoon butter, melted
- 2 tablespoons cream cheese
- 2 tablespoons coconut flour
- 1 tablespoon Swerve confectioners' style sweetener
- ½ teaspoon baking powder
- 1 medium egg
- ¼ teaspoon liquid stevia
- Drops vanilla extract
- Frozen raspberries

Directions:

1. Beat the butter with 2 tablespoons cream cheese in a mug, then place it in the microwave on high heat for about 1 minute until smooth.
2. Remove the mug from the microwave and let cool for 3 minutes.
3. Add the stevia, coconut flour, and baking powder, then mix again until the ingredients are well combined.
4. Add the Swerve, egg, and vanilla extract, and whisk while scraping down the sides of the mug. Put the frozen raspberries on top and press them into the mixture.
5. Again, bake in the microwave on high heat for 1 minute and 20 seconds until the top springs back lightly when gently pressed with your fingertip.
6. Remove from the microwave and cool for 5 minutes before serving.

Nutrition: Calories: 300 - Fat: 23.9g - Carbs: 12.1g - Fibre: 0.8g - Protein: 9.9g.

288. Spicy Almond Fat Bombs

Preparation time: 10 minutes
Cooking time: 4 minutes
Servings: 3
Ingredients:

- ¾ cup coconut oil
- ¼ cup almond butter
- ¼ cup cocoa powder
- Drops liquid stevia
- ⅛ teaspoon chilli powder

Special equipment:

- A 12-cup muffin pan

Directions:

1. Line a muffin pan with 12 paper liners. Keep aside.
2. Heat the oil in a small saucepan over low heat, then add the almond butter, cocoa powder, stevia, and chilli powder. Stir to combine well.
3. Divide the mixture evenly among the muffin cups and keep the muffin pan in the refrigerator for 15 minutes, or until the bombs are set and firm.
4. Serve immediately or refrigerate to chill until ready to serve.

Nutrition: Calories: 160 - Fat: 16.8g - Carbs: 2.0g Fibre: 1.2g - Protein: 1.5g.

289. Chocolate Granola Bars

Preparation time: 10 minutes
Cooking time: 20 minutes
Servings: 20
Ingredients:

- 3oz. almonds
- 3oz. walnuts
- 2oz. sesame seeds
- 2oz. pumpkin seeds
- 1oz. flaxseed
- 2oz. unsweetened coconut, shredded
- 2oz. dark chocolate with a minimum of 70% cocoa solids
- 2 tablespoons coconut oil
- 2 tablespoons tahini
- 1 teaspoon vanilla extract
- 2 teaspoons ground cinnamon
- 1 pinch sea salt
- 2 eggs

Directions:

1. Preheat your oven to 350°F.
2. Except for dark chocolate, process all the ingredients for granola in a food processor until they make a coarse and crumbly mixture.
3. Spread the granola mixture into a greased baking dish lined with parchment paper.
4. Bake the granola for 15 to 20 minutes in the oven until the cake turns golden brown.
5. Once baked, allow it to cool for 5 minutes, then remove from the baking dish.
6. Cut the granola cake into 24 bars using a sharp knife on a clean work surface. Set aside.
7. Melt the chocolate by heating in a double boiler or in the microwave. Let it cool for 5 minutes.
8. Serve the granola bars with the melted chocolate for dipping.

Nutrition: Calories: 145 - Fat: 17.2g - Carbs: 7.0g Fibre: 3.2g - Protein: 4.7g.

290. Coco Avocado Truffles

Preparation time: 35 minutes
Cooking time: 30 minutes
Servings: 10
Ingredients:

- 1 ripe avocado, chopped
- ½ teaspoon vanilla extract
- ½ lime zest
- 1 pinch salt
- 5oz. dark chocolate with a minimum of 80% cocoa solids, finely chopped
- 1 tablespoon coconut oil
- 1 tablespoon unsweetened cocoa powder

Directions:

1. In a bowl, thoroughly mix the avocado flesh with vanilla extract with an electric hand mixer until it forms a smooth mixture.
2. Add the lime zest and a pinch of salt, then mix well. Set aside.
3. Mix and melt the chocolate with coconut oil in a double broiler or by heating in the microwave.
4. Add the chocolate mixture to the avocado mash. Blend well until a smooth batter forms.
5. Refrigerate this batter for 30 minutes until firm.
6. Scoop portions of the batter (about 2 teaspoons in size) and shape into small truffle balls with your hands, then roll each truffle ball in the cocoa powder. Serve immediately.

Nutrition: Calories: 61 - Fat: 5.2g - Carbs: 4.3g - Fibre: 1.6g - Protein: 0.8g.

291.   Chocolate Peanut Fudge

Preparation time: 10 minutes
Cooking time: 35 minutes
Servings: 2
Ingredients:

- 3½ oz. dark chocolate with a minimum of 80% cocoa solids
- 2 tablespoons butter
- Pinch salt
- ¼ cup peanut butter
- ½ teaspoon vanilla extract
- 1 teaspoon ground cinnamon
- 1½ oz. salted peanuts, finely chopped

Directions:

1. Mix the chocolate with butter in a microwave-safe bowl, and heat in the microwave oven or in a double boiler to melt.
2. When the chocolate is melted, stir well until it is smooth, and leave the mixture to cool.
3. Mix well and add the remaining ingredients except for nuts, then stir to combine.
4. Transfer this chocolate batter to a greased baking pan lined with parchment paper.
5. Top the batter with peanuts and chill in the refrigerator for 2 hours until firm.
6. Remove from the refrigerator and cut into squares to serve.

Nutrition: Calories: 124 - Fat: 10.6g - Carbs: 5.9g Fibre: 1.6g - Protein: 2.9g.

292.   Pumpkin Spice Fat Bombs

Preparation Time: 10 minutes + 1 hours freezing
Cooking Time: 0 minutes
Servings: 16
Ingredients:

- ½ cup butter, at room temperature
- ½ cup cream cheese, at room temperature
- ⅓ cup pure pumpkin purée
- 2 tablespoons chopped almonds
- Drops liquid stevia
- ½ teaspoon ground cinnamon
- ¼ teaspoon ground nutmeg

Directions:

1. Line an 8-by-8-inch pan with parchment paper and set aside.
2. In a small bowl, whisk together the butter and cream cheese until very smooth.
3. Add the pumpkin purée and whisk until blended.
4. Stir in the almonds, stevia, cinnamon, and nutmeg.
5. Spoon the pumpkin mixture into the pan.
6. Use a spatula to spread it equally in the pan, then place it in the freezer for about 1 hour.
7. Cut into 16 pieces and store the fat bombs in a tightly sealed container in the freezer until ready to serve.

Nutrition: Calories: 87- Fat: 9g - Protein: 1g - Carbs: 1g - Fibre: 0g.

293.   Creamy Banana Fat Bombs

Preparation Time: 10 minutes + 1hour chilling
Cooking Time: 0 minutes
Servings: 4
Ingredients:

- 1¼ cups cream cheese, at room temperature
- ¾ cup heavy (whipping) cream
- 1 tablespoon pure banana extract
- Drops liquid stevia

Directions:

1. Line a baking sheet using parchment paper then set aside.
2. In a medium bowl, beat together the cream cheese, heavy cream, banana extract, and stevia until smooth and very thick, about 5 minutes.
3. Gently spoon the mixture onto the baking sheet in mounds, leaving some space between each mound, and place the baking sheet in the refrigerator until firm, about 1 hour.

Nutrition: Calories: 134 - Fat: 12g - Protein: 3g - Carbs: 1g - Fibre: 0g.

294. Nutty Shortbread Cookies

Preparation Time: 10 minutes + 30 minutes chilling
Cooking Time: 10 minutes
Servings: 18
Ingredients:
- ½ cup butter, plus for greasing the baking sheet
- ½ cup granulated sweetener
- 1 teaspoon alcohol-free pure vanilla extract
- 1½ cups almond flour
- ½ cup ground hazelnuts
- Pinch sea salt

Directions:
1. In a medium bowl, put and cream together the butter, sweetener, and vanilla until well blended.
2. Stir in the almond four, ground hazelnuts, and salt until a firm dough is formed.
3. Roll the dough into a 2-inch cylinder then wrap it using plastic wrap. Take the dough in the refrigerator for at least 30 minutes until firm.
4. Preheat the oven to 360°F. Line a baking sheet with parchment paper and lightly grease the paper with butter; set aside.
5. Unwrap the chilled cylinder, slice the dough into 18 cookies, and place the cookies on the baking sheet.
6. Bake the cookies up to firm and lightly browned, about 10 minutes.
7. Allow the cookies to cool on the baking sheet for 5-6 minutes and then transfer them to a wire rack to cool completely.

Nutrition: Calories: 105 - Fat: 10g Carbs: 2g - Protein: 3g - Fibre: 1g.

295. Intermittent Lava Cake

Preparation time: 15 minutes
Cooking time: 10 minutes
Servings: 6
Ingredients:
- Melted butter, for greasing the ramekins
- 2oz. dark chocolate with a min. of 70% cocoa solids
- 2oz. butter
- ¼ teaspoon vanilla extract
- 2 eggs

Special equipment:
- 6 small ramekins

Directions:
1. Preheat your oven to 370°F and lightly grease 4 to 6 small ramekins with 1 tablespoon melted butter.
2. Cut the chocolate into small pieces on your cutting board. Add the chocolate and butter to a double broiler, and heat until they are melted. Mix well.
3. Add the vanilla to the chocolate mixture, then allow the mixture to cool.
4. Beat all the eggs in a mixing bowl for 3 minutes until fluffy, then add the chocolate mixture. Stir to combine.
5. Divide the mixture among the greased ramekins. Bake all the ramekins in the preheated oven for 5 minutes.
6. Remove from the oven and cool for 5 minutes before enjoying.

Nutrition: Calories: 197 - Fat: 17.8g - Carbs: 5g Protein: 5.4g - Fibre: 1.0g.

296. Spiced Chocolate Fat Bombs

Preparation Time: 10 minutes + 15 minutes chilling
Cooking Time: 4 minutes
Servings: 12
Ingredients:

- ¾ cup coconut oil
- ¼ cup cocoa powder
- ¼ cup almond butter
- ⅛ teaspoon chilli powder
- Drops liquid stevia

Directions:

1. Line a mini muffin tin using paper liners and set aside.
2. Put a small saucepan over low heat and add the coconut oil, cocoa powder, almond butter, chilli powder, and stevia.
3. Heat until the coconut oil is melted, and then whisk to blend.
4. Spoon the mixture into the muffin cups and place the tin in the refrigerator until the bombs are firm about 15 minutes.
5. Transfer the cups to an airtight container and store the fat bombs in the freezer until you want to serve them.

Nutrition: Calories: 117 - Fat: 12g - Protein: 2g - Carbs: 2g - Fibre: 0g.

297. Vanilla Almond Ice Pops

Preparation Time: 10 minutes + 4 hours chilling
Cooking Time: 15 minutes
Servings: 18
Ingredients:

- 2 cups almond milk
- 1 cup heavy (whipping) cream
- 1 vanilla bean, halved lengthwise
- 1 cup shredded unsweetened coconut

Directions:

7. Set a medium saucepan on medium heat, then put the almond milk, heavy cream, and vanilla bean.
8. Bring the liquid to a simmer and reduce the heat to low. Continue to simmer for 5 minutes.
9. Remove the saucepan from the heat and let the liquid cool.
10. Take the vanilla bean out of the liquid and use a knife to scrape the seeds out of the bean into the liquid.
11. Stir in the coconut and divide the liquid between the ice pop molds.
12. Freeze until solid, about 4 hours, and enjoy.

Nutrition: Calories: 166 - Fat: 15g - Protein: 3g - Carbs: 4g - Fibre: 2g.

298. Snickerdoodles

Preparation Time: 10 minutes
Cooking Time: 10 minutes
Servings: 18
Ingredients:

- 1 ½ cups almond flour
- 2 tablespoons butter
- ½ cup + 2 tablespoons Sukrin Gold
- 1 egg
- 1 teaspoon pure vanilla extract
- ¼ teaspoon salt
- ¼ teaspoon ground cinnamon
- ¼ teaspoon ground nutmeg
- ⅛ teaspoon ground cloves

Directions:

1. Preheat your oven to 350°F.
2. Line cookie sheets with parchment paper.
3. In a bowl, mix the almond flour, Sukrin, and salt together.
4. Add in butter, vanilla, and egg.
5. Roll dough into 18 balls.
6. In another bowl, mix 2 tablespoons Sukrin with spices.
7. Roll cookies in it to coat.
8. Arrange on the cookie sheets.
9. Bake for 8 minutes, then check. If the sides are starting to brown and the middle looks cooked, they are done. If not, bake another 2 minutes.
10. Cool before serving!

Nutrition: Total Calories: 94 Carbs: 2g - Fat: 9g - Protein: 2g - Fibre: 0g.

299. Mascarpone Berry Parfait

Preparation Time: 5 minutes
Cooking Time: 0 minutes
Servings: 12
Ingredients:
- ⅓ pint raspberries
- ⅓ pint strawberries
- ⅓ pint blueberries
- 8oz. mascarpone cheese
- 1 cup heavy whipping cream
- ¾ teaspoon liquid stevia
- 1 teaspoon pure vanilla extract

Directions:
1. Whip cream, mascarpone, stevia, and vanilla in a bowl until you get stiff, fluffy peaks.
2. Spoon into serving cups and mix in berries.

Nutrition: Calories: 159 - Protein: 2g - Carbs: 3g Fat: 17g - Fibre: 0g.

300. Macadamia Brownies

Preparation Time: 20 minutes
Cooking Time: 40 minutes
Servings: 20
Ingredients:
- 9oz. unsalted butter
- 4 ½ oz. dark cooking chocolate
- 2 cups castor sugar
- 4 whole eggs
- 1 teaspoon vanilla extract
- 1 cup plain (all purpose) flour
- 1/4 cup cocoa powder
- 1/2 teaspoon salt
- 4 ½oz. toasted macadamia nuts

Directions:
1. Preheat oven to 355°F. on bake, not fan
2. Line a baking dish with parchment paper. (10 ½ inch x 7 inch)
3. Melt butter over low heat
4. When butter is half melted add the chocolate, stir till completely melted and combined
5. Remove pan from heat and whisk in sugar
6. Beat in eggs one at a time until mixture is shiny
7. Stir in vanilla
8. Sift in flour, cocoa and salt and mix till combined
9. Stir through macadamia nuts
10. Bake for 35-40 minutes or till a skewer comes out clean
11. Remove from oven and place tin on a cake rack to cool
12. Lift brownie onto a chopping board and slice into pieces
13. Serve and enjoy!

Nutrition: Calories: 230 - Protein: 2g - Carbs: 22g - Fat: 15g - Fibre: 1g.

301. Rum Chocolate Pralines

Preparation Time: 10 minutes + chilling time
Cooking Time: 0 minutes
Servings: 8
Ingredients:
- 1 cup bakers' chocolate, sugar-free
- 2 tablespoons dark rum
- 1/8 teaspoon ground cloves
- 1/8 teaspoon cinnamon powder
- 1/2 teaspoon almond extract
- 1/2 teaspoon rum extract
- 2 tablespoons cocoa powder
- 1/4 cup almond butter
- 1 cup almond milk

Directions:
1. Microwave the chocolate, cocoa, and almond butter until they have completely melted.
2. Add in the other ingredients and mix to combine well. Pour the mixture into silicone molds and place them in your refrigerator until set.

Nutrition: Calories: 70 - Fat: 3.4g - Carbs: 5.1g - Protein: 2.4g - Fibre: 1.6g.

302. Intermittent Cacao Butter Blondies

Preparation Time: 15 minutes
Cooking Time: 20 minutes
Servings: 20
Ingredients:

- 6 tablespoons cacao butter
- ½ cup erythritol (powdered)
- 4 tablespoons unsalted butter (softened, room temperature)
- ¼ teaspoon baking powder
- 2 pieces large eggs (room temperature)
- ¼ cup almond flour
- 2 tablespoons coconut flour
- 2 tablespoons coconut cream
- 2 tablespoons walnuts (ground)
- ½oz. dark chocolate (chopped)
- 1 teaspoon vanilla bean seeds
- 1 teaspoon vanilla extract
- 1 pinch stevia extract
- 1 dash salt

Directions:

1. Preheat your oven to 360°F. Prepare a square baking pan (8") and line it with parchment paper.
2. In a microwave-safe mixing bowl, put in the cacao butter. Microwave it for 90 seconds to melt. Stir the melted butter and make sure that there are no more lumps in it. Microwave again to melt the lumps, if needed. Let it cool completely.
3. Once the melted cacao butter is cooled, mix in the unsalted butter and stir.
4. In another mixing bowl, put in the eggs, vanilla bean seeds, vanilla extract, erythritol, and salt. Mix them well for 2 minutes using an electric hand mixer.
5. Put in the coconut cream into the egg mixture. Mix well.
6. Put in the cooled melted cacao butter mixture into the egg mixture. Continue mixing until the consistency gets dense.
7. In another mixing bowl, sift the almond flour, coconut flour, and baking powder. Mix well.
8. Pour the flour mixture into the cream mixture. Mix well.
9. Put in the chopped chocolate and ground walnuts. Mix well.
10. Transfer the batter into the lined baking pan. Spread out the batter evenly on the baking pan.
11. Bake the batter for 20 minutes. Do not over-bake it. Do the toothpick test to know that it is the right time to take the blondies out from the oven.
12. Carefully take out the entire batch of blondies from the pan, including the parchment paper. Put it on the rack to cool down.
13. Once completely cooled, cut into 20 blondie squares. It is recommended to leave the blondies overnight on the counter before serving.

Nutrition: Calories: 80 - Carbs: 1.6g - Fat: 7.3g - Protein: 2.1g - Fibre: 0.9g.

303. Delicious Coffee Ice Cream

Preparation Time: 10 minutes
Cooking Time: 5 minutes
Servings: 1
Ingredients:

- 3oz. coconut cream, frozen into ice cubes
- 1 ripe avocado, diced and frozen
- ½ cup coffee expresso
- ½ tbsp. sweetener
- 1 tsp vanilla extract
- 1 tbsp. water
- Coffee beans

Directions:

1. Take out the frozen coconut cubes and avocado from the fridge. Slightly melt them for 5-10 minutes.
2. Add the sweetener, coffee expresso, and vanilla extract to the coconut-avocado mix and whisk with an immersion blender until it becomes creamy (for about 1 minute). Pour in the water and blend for 30 seconds.
3. Top with coffee beans and enjoy!

Nutrition: Calories: 596 - Carbs: 20.5g - Fat: 61g Protein: 6.3g.

Thanks for reading this far!

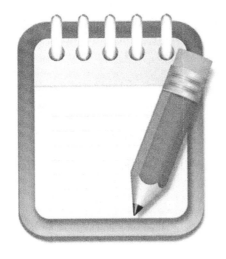 I would be grateful if you could take a minute of your time to leave an honest Amazon review about my work, so that we can share your experience with other customers.

Thanks again!

 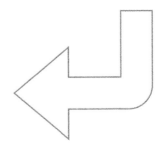

Conclusion

Intermittent fasting is an optimal tool to lead a healthy life. By following the principles of intermittent fasting you can surely reach your goal of healthy and disease-free life. However, you must not see intermittent fasting just as a way to shed your extra pounds. Because intermittent fasting is not just a dieting method, it is a way of life.

Your body is a gift, and you need to take care of it. Excessive weight and obesity are surely health issues that must be dealt properly. And one of the right ways is intermittent fasting. Everyone has their capacity. Everybody is different with different needs and perspectives. This is the reason why intermittent fasting may not work for all of you. Therefore, you all must evaluate your body needs and stamina before setting on the journey of intermittent fasting. The intermittent fasting method is suitable for some people while for others it is not the right answer. You need to find out which category you belong to.

The most important thing to keep in mind while starting intermittent fasting is that you don't need to overburden yourself. As this is not a matter of few days or few weeks. You have to adopt that method, which you can continue in the long run with the same consistency. Intermittent fasting is a lifestyle. So you have to adopt this lifestyle and get used to it. No one changes their lifestyle now and then. Start following this method, if you don't feel good about it, you can leave any time. The body is yours hence the choice is all yours. However, don't jump to the conclusion hastily. You need to wait for a few days for results to show up. You will surely see positive changes in your body and mental health. Our bodies are designed in a way that they can adapt to the changes pretty quickly. You just need to train your body and mind to continue the process. Once your body gets the hang of it there is no turning around. But if the method is not working for you, you can surely look for other alternatives out there.

Another important thing to keep in mind is the way you follow intermittent fasting. This method is all about restricting your mealtime around a certain period. So you must eat healthy and nutritious food during the eating time. A lot of people don't like the idea of and think that it is difficult to follow. The answer to this problem is that fasting is surely difficult at the start but not impossible. Indolent and unhealthy lifestyle is at peak these days. We all spend our time, watching television, or scrolling through our phones. Our active time is much shorter that leads to body issues like weight gain and sometimes serious health problems like cardiac problems or diabetes. These problems can be overcome with the intermittent fasting method, in which not only, you have to restrict your meals, but also do regular exercise. In conclusion, you are in charge of your body, so you must make the best decision regarding your body, mind, and health.

Made in the USA
Monee, IL
13 October 2022

15785239R00085